PLANET
HEAL THYSELF

DESTINY IMAGE BOOKS BY JORDAN RUBIN

The Maker's Diet

The Maker's Diet Revolution

The Maker's Diet Transformation DVD

The Maker's Diet Transformation Journal

Maker's Diet Meals

The Joseph Blessing

PLANET
HEAL THYSELF

The REVOLUTION *of*
REGENERATION
in BODY, MIND, *and* PLANET

JORDAN RUBIN

DESTINY IMAGE® PUBLISHERS, INC.
P.O. Box 310, Shippensburg, PA 17257-0310
"Promoting Inspired Lives."

This book and all other Destiny Image and Destiny Image Fiction books are available at Christian bookstores and distributors worldwide.

Cover design by: Eileen Rockwell

For more information on foreign distributors, call 717-532-3040.
Reach us on the Internet: www.destinyimage.com.

ISBN 13 TP: 978-0-7684-0859-1
ISBN 13 eBook: 978-0-7684-0860-7

For Worldwide Distribution, Printed in the U.S.A.
2 3 4 5 6 7 8 / 20 19 18 17 16

FSC Printed on FSC Certified paper

Contents

INTRODUCTION   The Revolution of Regeneration 7

1.   The Circle of Life: Real Nutrients from
     Real Foods Create Real Health 23

2.   Sprouting to Life 41

3.   Fantastic Fermentation. 53

4.   Eat Organic 75

5.   Say No to GMO 97

6.   Go Gluten-Free 115

7.   The Power of Plants 129

8.   Avoid Eight Common Allergens 159

9.   Become an Artisanal Eater. 177

10. Heal the Planet: Living the Eco-Regenerative Lifestyle 189

     Source Material 245

Introduction

The Revolution of Regeneration

I FOUND OUT WHAT IT WAS LIKE TO LIVE IN A DEGENERATING BODY when I was nineteen years old.

I didn't have a well-known autoimmune disease such as multiple sclerosis or ALS, serious neurological disorders that worsen over time. Nor was I stricken with leukemia, a form of cancer that affects the body's ability to make healthy blood cells and is one of the most common cancers for teenagers and young adults.

What was sending me on a lonely path toward a seemingly certain and untimely death was an inflammatory bowel disease known as Crohn's disease—the worst case they'd ever seen, my doctors said. What this meant in practical terms was that my body was breaking down because of my digestive tract's disharmony and massive inflammation as well as its inability to convert food into energy and assimilate basic nutrients to feed the entire body.

I was an unlikely casualty of a broken system of degeneration—a college kid who'd just finished his freshman year at Florida State University, eager to experience the world and embrace life. I really believed I had a sunny future and that my best days were on the horizon, but suddenly, out of nowhere, my body started deteriorating rapidly. In a matter of days, I went from being the picture of good health to a scared, confused, and emotionally battered young man who couldn't believe how swiftly his life had changed.

Following the spring semester of my freshman year, I came home and hung out with friends for a few weeks before I had to report to a summer camp as a counselor. This is when the deterioration of my health began.

Out of nowhere, I was hit with nausea, stomach cramps, high fever, and horrible digestive problems. I thought I was fighting a nasty bug, but I didn't rebound like I usually did. This first wave of discomfort was followed by a tsunami of violent and bloody diarrhea that knocked me for a loop and sapped any remaining energy I had. I dropped twenty pounds from my already lean frame in just six days at camp.

I hung on as long as I could because I didn't want to come to grips with my rapidly deteriorating health. I didn't have the appetite for the "camp chow," so the lack of nutritional sustenance took its toll as well. What little I managed to eat resulted in painful cramps, high fever, and more brutal diarrhea. I had to always know where the nearest bathroom was in case I had to do the "penguin walk." After another week of misery, I couldn't function. I had to go home.

A friend drove me back to my hometown of Palm Beach Gardens in South Florida, where Mom took me to my family doctor. He poked and prodded my abdomen, then ran a battery of tests that all came back negative. Just before leaving the examination room, my doctor wrote me a prescription for two antibiotics. "You'll be okay," he promised. "I don't see any reason why you can't go back to school this fall."

I rallied barely enough to return for the fall semester, but my time in Tallahassee turned out to be a disaster. My physical strength ebbed. Just before midterms, I had to withdraw from school and come home. This time around, we all knew it was *serious*. When my fever spiked to 105 degrees one night, Mom and Dad immediately stepped into action, filling our bathtub with ice and cold water, but I was close to incoherent.

My parents rushed me to the local hospital, where specialists and medical technicians conducted various tests, including a sigmoidoscopy and an upper GI series that allowed them to examine the condition of my intestinal tract. They were looking for any irregularities.

I was examined by a gastroenterologist, who recognized the symptoms of high fever, night sweats, loss of appetite, general feeling of weakness, severe abdominal cramps, and diarrhea—often bloody—as symptoms of inflammatory bowel disease. After running a battery of diagnostic tests, the doctor delivered a stunning verdict: I was stricken with a digestive ailment known as Crohn's disease.

"How do we treat it?" I asked.

"There's no known cure," replied the gastroenterologist. "You'll probably be on powerful anti-inflammatory and immunosuppressives for the rest of your life. You could be facing surgery to remove parts of your small intestine and potentially your entire colon."

To a nineteen-year-old preparing to find his way in the world, that sounded like a fate worse than death.

A ROUGH ROAD

I couldn't believe the news. I immediately fell into despair.

I seemed like one of the most unlikely young adults to be struck down in my prime because my parents, Herb and Phyllis Rubin, were two of the most health-minded people you'd ever meet. They'd done everything they could to raise me in a healthy manner, especially in the area of diet.

My father was a naturopathic physician and chiropractor who sought a more natural approach in treating patients and their aches and pains. Mom was a back-to-nature type as well who filled her cupboards with raw honey, wheat germ, and lentils and stocked our refrigerator with homemade soy milk, sprouts, and tofu. She didn't allow fried chips and store-bought cookies in the house, which made me just about the least popular kid in the neighborhood.

So when I became deathly ill at the age of nineteen, my parents were very proactive. Over the next year and a half, they would take me to sixty-nine doctors, natural practitioners, and health experts from every spectrum of the medical world—from conventional medicine to alternative and experimental therapies. During a two-year period, I read more than three hundred books on health and nutrition. You name the diet, you name the nutritional supplement, I tried it. I left no stone unturned.

Nothing stopped the death spiral that my health was in. I lost nearly half of my body weight and was reduced to 104 pounds, a frightfully thin figure who resembled a concentration camp victim. My medical team told my parents to hope for the best but be prepared for the worst.

I'll never forget the night in my hospital room when nurses, phlebotomists, and doctors desperately tried to get an IV in me to rehydrate my shriveled body. After one failed attempt, a nurse ran out of my hospital room. I overheard her say, "This young man isn't going to make it through the night."

I truly believed this was it for me. I had made peace with God and was ready to die. After four hours of agony, though, they successfully inserted a needle into my vein.

I woke up the next morning alive, but I was far from healed. When my condition stabilized, I was sent home with a half-dozen medications to deal with the stabbing pains in my gut, and I made dozens of trips to the bathroom each day.

It was about that time when I lifted a special prayer to God. "Lord, if you heal me and I come out of this alive," I prayed, "and if I can help just one person overcome a horrific disease like mine, this living hell will have all been worth it."

I also took a major step of faith by asking my mother to take a picture in my emaciated condition.

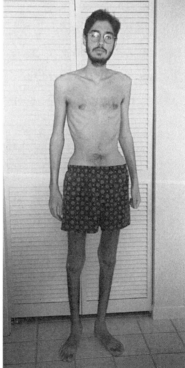

"You really think that's a good idea?" she asked. "Maybe we should wait until you get better."

"No, Mom. This is something I really want to do. Someday, I want the world to see the miracle that's about to happen in my life."

With great reluctance, she grabbed her camera. I stood in our hallway, wearing glasses and a pair of boxer shorts as well as a look of resignation. I had a beard because I was too weak to shave and couldn't afford to nick myself with my unsteady hand. I weighed 111 pounds that morning and stood on legs that resembled worn toothpicks.

My stomach was as gaunt as someone in a Third World country experiencing starvation.

Mom snapped the photo, and then I slumped back into bed, too tired to stand any longer.

My health continued to degenerate. The medical doctors counseled my parents that it was time for me to go under the knife. My only hope, they said, was for me to go to Mount Sinai Hospital in New York City for a procedure that would remove my large intestine and part of my small intestine. Or, if I wanted to chance it, I could undergo an experimental (at the time) operation called a "J-pouch" in which my colon would be removed and a reservoir would be constructed from the small intestine to collect the body's waste products.

Once my abdomen was sliced open and my large intestine was cut out and removed, there was no turning back. I would forever live a compromised existence. With what little fight I had left in me, I stalled for time because once I boarded a flight for New York City, I was out of options.

Then, a ray of light. My father, in a desperate attempt to stave off my surgery, heard about a San Diego nutritionist named Bud Keith who had helped people in desperate straits like myself. Dad got his phone number and called him, and during their first conversation, Bud offered to show me a health plan found in the pages of the Bible, proven through history and confirmed by science. He believed I could be healed if I followed his recommendations.

I had nothing to lose. It was either fly to San Diego and give it a shot or book a flight to New York City and go the radical surgery route. As I prayed for guidance, I believed that traveling west was the direction I needed go. I was confident that this was the plan for me.

At the Palm Beach International Airport, I had to be rolled down the Jetway in a wheelchair to board my flight. Upon my arrival in San Diego, Bud Keith was there to greet me and take me under his wing. He showed me what foods to eat, taught me to forgive and let go of my past hurts, and trust that my healing was coming soon.

Then a miracle happened. After forty days, I added twenty-nine much-needed pounds and topped 150 pounds for the first time in nearly two years. In six more weeks, my body *totally* regenerated, and I was ready to begin my life again.

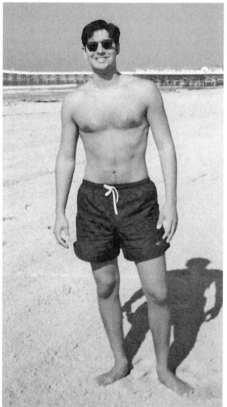

Not only did I get well without medication or surgery, but I was inspired with a passion to transform the health of this nation and world one life at a time. Upon returning home to South Florida, I worked at a health food store where I shared my story and encouraged many customers to change their diet. A few short months later, I started a health and nutrition company and wrote about my experiences in a book called *Patient Heal Thyself,* followed by a *New York Times* best-selling book called *The Maker's Diet.* In total, the two books have more than 3 million copies in print.

Having a best-selling book like *The Maker's Diet* opened doors to share my life-changing experiences throughout America as well as spanning the globe. I was interviewed by the major media—television, radio, magazine, and newspapers. I hosted an international television program and began writing more books on nutrition, health, and wellness. I married Nicki, and we became parents. Our first child, a son named Joshua, came to us naturally, but since then we've felt led to adopt *five* children. Life has been incredibly busy.

In 2009, Nicki and I purchased thousands of acres of Missouri farmland that was certified organic one year later. Taking nutrition a step "beyond organic" has been a longtime passion of mine that has resulted in a focused mission to provide people with the world's healthiest foods and beverages. Who would have ever thought that a nineteen-year-old on death's door would be thrust into what could be the most important crossroads the world has ever experienced?

I certainly didn't, which is why I feel a calling to tell others that what's happening to our bodies mirrors what's happening to the planet. Everywhere I look, I see people living lives with compromised health and great suffering. Everywhere I travel, I see our environment in utter disarray and in need of healing.

In today's day and age, we are simply pushing our bodies and the planet beyond the brink, asking our bodies and our planet to function properly amidst tremendous environmental damage that we are inflicting on ourselves and the world around us. We expect more and provide less—much less. The nutrition our bodies need is simply not being supplied. Likewise, the nutrients in our soil are disappearing at an alarming rate. In an effort to put back what we've lost, we fortify our foods with a few synthetic "vitamins" and supply our soil with a few synthetic "minerals."

In order to combat the degenerating health of our bodies, we consume massive amounts of medications, including antibiotics, to "kill" the germs that medical scientists believe are causing diseases, but we weaken our already battered digestive tracts and immune systems.

We use pesticides to kill the insects that agricultural scientists believe are destroying our crops, but our plants may be susceptible due to their weakened and hybridized state.

Today's residents of Earth have been born into a system of degeneration that harms the planet and every person and creature alive in this day and age. In order to see the transformation we desire, we must "opt out" of the modern systems of degeneration, including medicine, agriculture, and education. When I say "opt out," I don't necessarily mean for you to never see a doctor, avoid consuming foods found in a grocery store, and homeschool your children. I simply want you to understand that the health and well-being of you, your family, and our planet rests on your shoulders and the daily decisions you make. Few people understand that our bodies as well as our land are degenerating rapidly, but the statistics are clear. The path is here, and it's time for you and me to take the first step toward regeneration.

It's time for us to join together and help the planet and its people *heal thyself.*

BUILDING FROM THE GROUND UP

Ever since I was healed nearly twenty years ago, I've studied under some of the greatest minds in medicine, nutrition, and sustainable agriculture. I've gotten my hands dirty raising fruits, vegetables, cattle, sheep, goats, chickens, and bees on our organic farm.

If my old friends at Palm Beach Gardens High could see me now.

When my family and I moved from Florida to our farm in Southern Missouri in 2013, I noticed wide swaths of land where the topsoil was totally gone. I decided to do something about it by instituting a holistic grazing program and constructing a soil-building composting area near the chicken coops to make healthy topsoil. Each day, manure waste from our organic dairy is brought over by loaders and mixed with untreated oak wood chips. The kids carry buckets of food waste from our kitchen—eggshells, banana peels, orange rinds, etc.—that they dump in the area. Roaming chickens hunt and peck through the food scraps, adding their own manure. Mix it all up, and you have the makings of healthy dirt that we're spreading around the farm.

Even though what we're doing to restore our farmland is just a blip on the radar screen, I want to do my part to heal the planet because when we talk about the future of our ecosystem and all the animals and plants, everything depends on the health of our soil—particularly topsoil.

Bill Wilson, founder of Midwest Permaculture, raised my consciousness on topsoil. Permaculture is an amalgamation of two words: *permanent culture*. This phrase refers to a system where all humans live well and we leave the planet in better condition than we found it. Permaculture is a creative and artful way of living, where people and nature are preserved and enhanced by thoughtful planning, careful use of natural resources, and a respectful approach for life.

The way we farm today is *not* permanent or sustainable but industrial and mechanized to maximize production—good for the short term but devastating in the long run. The way we do agriculture has resulted in topsoil depletion and groundwater contamination, increased pesticide resistance, and contributed to the disintegration of economic and social conditions in rural areas.

In addition, the system of monocrop agriculture—growing the same crop on the same land year after year—may produce bushels of wheat and soybeans, but the price is more degeneration for the planet. First of all, the pests and insects—who know they can return at the same time each year for something to munch on—are becoming more and more genetically resistant to pesticides, herbicides, and fungicides needed to fend them off. Second, when crops are not rotated, the soil's nutrients are depleted like chips in a losing poker game—slowly but surely.

In addition, commercial farmers raising crops inorganically utilize synthetic fertilizers to stimulate rapid plant growth, but these fertilizers are made up of nitrogen salts, combined with phosphorus and potassium known as NPK, which provides imbalanced nutrition at best to the soil. That's another reason why the nutritive value of foods grown in these soils has declined significantly in the last hundred years. When Americans are subsisting on a diet of nutrient-poor foods of both plant and animal origin, it's no surprise that our health is degenerating.

Let's take a closer look at why we are losing our topsoil. Bill Wilson of Midwest Permaculture pointed out that his home state of Illinois has some of the richest soil in the world. Back in 1850 or so, the humus (also called soil organic matter) content of Illinois soil was between 10 and 13 percent, which was normal for native soils in North America. Humus refers to the organic matter—leaves, worm casings, tree branches, tree limbs, and dead animals—that has fallen into the soil and decomposed over time. Humus provides food for the soil's bacteria and gives soil its spongy feel because of the way it holds moisture.

Today, Illinois' farmlands have a humus content of 1.3 percent, which is a dramatic loss but still one of the highest levels in the country. Most soils across America have a humus content of 1 percent. The reason these numbers are significant is because we need at least 3 percent for biological activity to exist in the soil; otherwise there is not enough food for most of the biology to happen.

Our soil's humus content has dropped so precipitously because of the way we "turn over" the soil each year. Every time the farmer's massive plowing machines break open the soil to create a seed bed, they are exposing the soil to air—meaning they are dumping oxygen into the soil. When that happens during the plowing process, the bacteria count shoots way up and increases rapidly—and consumes humus. When farmers add in herbicides and fertilizers, that accelerates the killing of all sorts of microbiology in the soil.

The upshot of all this activity is that our fields produce smaller crops: corn stalks and soybeans don't grow as high and yellow in the middle in the summer. But that's the least of our worries compared to how fast our topsoil is *disappearing.*

You don't hear about topsoil erosion or vanishing grasslands very much these days, but we should because disappearing dirt could rival climate change as an environmental threat. Topsoil is the "thin brown line"—a shallow skin of nutrient-rich matter—that grows our food and plays a crucial role in supporting life on Earth.

"We're losing more and more of it every day," said David Montgomery, a University of Washington geologist. "The estimate is that we are losing about 1 percent of our topsoil every year to erosion, most of this caused by modern agriculture." Up until the start of the 20th century, topsoil was twelve inches deep, on average. Today, it's maybe six inches deep.

I've heard estimates that if soil depletion continues at this rate, we have between sixty and two hundred years of decent farming left before our fields turn into arid, dusty plots of land. Once topsoil's gone, it's really hard to bring it back. To maintain topsoil, fields must lie fallow every few years, crops must be rotated, and measures must be taken to prevent water and wind erosion.

People forget that topsoil is living material and that in every handful of dirt, there are trillions of beneficial microorganisms necessary for our digestive health. These microbes are responsible for a cycle of life by making the soil more resilient and able to hold moisture, but that cycle gets interrupted when nutrients are lost from the soil. That happens from overgrazing, from tilling the soil after every harvest, and from burning off the stubble in the field to make the next crop easier to plant.

Bill Wilson points out that the number-one export in the United States is not corn, wheat, or oil but…topsoil. Much of it ends up in our major rivers, such as the mighty Mississippi, where if you took a gallon of water at the mouth of the Mississippi and measured the suspended solids, you'd have a significant amount of dirt. In fact, every three to ten seconds, depending upon the season of the year, a truckload of topsoil reaches the mouth of the Mississippi. A couple of billion tons of dirt erodes from U.S. land each year.

Lest you're not convinced that the planet needs to heal thyself, may I remind you about the "cradle of civilization"—the convergence of the Tigris and Euphrates rivers that became known as Mesopotamia but is comprised today of modern-day Iraq, Kuwait, and the northeastern section of Syria. Thousands of years ago, the "Fertile Crescent" was comprised of rich farmlands teeming with topsoil that supported civilization's first cities. Today, a more apt name would be the Not-So-Fertile Crescent because extensive damming of the two rivers and the heavy draining of the river basin has obliterated the topsoil.

People I've talked to say that the same dust bowl scenario can happen here unless steps are taken to end the degeneration of our most precious natural resource—the nutrient-rich soil used to grow our fruits, vegetables, and grains.

Our permaculture manager on our organic farm read me an amazing quote from Vigen Gurolan, author of *The Fragrance of God*, that bears repeating here: "God created humankind so that humankind might cultivate the earthly and thereby create the heavenly."

I speak from experience when I say that regenerative farming certainly brings one closer to God.

DEFINITELY NOT THE HIGHWAY TO HEALTH

Like tons and tons of muddy water working its way down the Mississippi River, millions and millions don't realize their health is moving slowly toward a day of reckoning either.

An entire planet of people needs to heal thyself.

Take cancer for starters. Males have one-in-two chance of developing cancer in their lifetime and a one-in-four chance of dying from the disease, according to the American Cancer Society. Women are a bit better off: they have a one-in-three chance of developing cancer including a one-in-five chance of dying from breast, ovarian, or other types of cancers.

As grim as these odds are, heart disease and stroke are the leading causes of death and disability in the United States. Diabetes, gallbladder disease, liver disease, and osteoarthritis are other afflictions leading to pain and suffering and shortened life expectancy. Autoimmune diseases are being diagnosed in record numbers. Childhood diseases are on the rise as well. It's an ugly picture of degeneration.

So let's review what I've discussed up to this point. When I was born, there was the expectation that I would grow up healthy and live a long, vibrant life, just like anyone else. At the age of nineteen, however, I became a casualty of the modern system of degeneration.

I survived through God's grace, and ever since, I feel compelled to help others overcome their health challenges. As I look around, though, I see how the civilized areas of our planet are falling prey to the modern scourge of degeneration that we're all born into. We must take deliberate steps to improve our health and save our planet.

The underlying theme of *Planet Heal Thyself* is that our bodies mirror the degeneration happening all over our planet and we must "reverse the curse," if you will. The advent of modern agriculture and modern medicine has done wonders to feed billions and extend our life expectancy, but many of the practices employ a robbing-Peter-to-pay-Paul mentality that does not bode well for our future or the future of our children.

So what can we, as individuals, do to fix this system of degeneration that impacts each and every one of us?

A lot more than you think, and you can start by following the Get Real 10—ten important steps or standards that will guide you as a productive citizen of planet Earth and a consumer of goods to feed yourself, which I will lay out in the following pages of *Planet Heal Thyself.*

These are ten steps that you can employ with the selfish goal (okay, not so selfish when you consider how important you are to so many people) to improve the health of your body and, by virtue of that, begin to transform the health of our planet simultaneously. In the following chapters, I will unpack each of the Get Real 10 promises listed below:

1. Eat real food.

2. Eat sprouted food.

3. Eat fermented food.

4. Eat organically grown and raised food.

5. Say no to foods that are genetically altered/containing GMOs.

6. Eat gluten-free.

7. Eat an abundance of plant-based foods.

8. Avoid and/or minimize eight common allergens in your diet.

9. Eat foods that are handcrafted or artisanal.

10. Purchase foods and other consumable items that are housed in eco-regenerative packaging, lightening the environmental impact on our planet and contributing to future soil building.

Please know at the outset that I practice what I preach, meaning if you came to my farm or visited my home, you'd see me following the Get Real 10 promises. But I'm also putting my mouth where my heart is. A small group of merry men, women, and myself have created the Heal the Planet Farm and the Heal the Planet Foundation within our Beyond Organic ranch. Our goal is to take several hundred certified organic acres and begin to heal the land by building topsoil, using permaculture, and employing holistic management and polycultural techniques of regenerative agriculture. By doing so, we can devote much of what we produce to feed and build our soil as well as feed and build up the local impoverished community. Now this is what I call a win-win.

We want to do our part to heal the planet and its people. We're going to stop feeding chemicals to our children and the land and give back what they need, and we're going to do that for the world to see. It's time to regenerate and stop sustaining what's not working.

If you want to take the first step toward joining the revolution of regeneration, welcome aboard. As they say, the journey of a 1,000 steps begins with a single one. If you want to make a difference and see real transformation in your body and our planet, please read on!

1

The Circle of Life: Real Nutrients from Real Foods Create Real Health

WITH SIX CHILDREN UNDER OUR ROOF, AND ALL BUT ONE UNDER THE age of twelve, we gravitate toward G-rated movies whenever the kids watch videos.

A perennial favorite is *The Lion King*, the animated Disney classic that was released twenty years ago. This heroic coming-of-age story follows the epic adventures of a young lion cub named Simba who struggles to accept the responsibilities of growing up and coming to grips with his destined role as king of the jungle.

Simba's father is King Mufasa, the revered ruler of the animal kingdom. As a father, Mufasa feels that it's important to teach his son about the "Circle of Life," or the delicate balance of nature that bonds all animals together. Early in the movie, Mufasa and Simba are walking through the savannah when they have this conversation:

Mufasa: Everything you see exists together, in a delicate balance. As king, you need to understand that balance, and respect all the creatures—from the crawling ant to the leaping antelope.

Simba: But, Dad, don't we eat the antelope?

Mufasa: Yes, Simba, but let me explain. When we die, our bodies become the grass. And the antelope eat the grass. And so we are all connected in the great Circle of Life.

The Circle of Life applies to the humans inhabiting this planet as well, although we don't have any natural predators and the chance of being eaten by killer whales, sharks, crocodiles, tigers, and, yes, lions is beyond miniscule. Even though we're at the top of the food chain, we are highly dependent on what's beneath us—all the way to the ground. And it's from the ground where real foods receive real nutrients to create real health.

Just as the savannah—a grassy plain in tropical and subtropical regions—supports the antelope and lion alike and all creatures in between, the soil on our farms and ranches provides the nutrients that we need to survive. Our existence is dependent upon thriving, living topsoil, which is made of composted materials that become humus over time, or what we call soil organic matter (SOM).

Soil organic matter is a component of soil made from the cells and tissues of plants and animal residues at various stages of decomposition. Or, looked at another way, soil organic matter is the amount of organic compounds in the soil that is not clay or rock. When you have the right percentage of soil organic matter in dirt, you've got real nutrition for the planet because the soil organic matter provides food for the microbes that builds and/or maintains the health of topsoil. Not everyone thinks about our relationship with the soil, but the real "circle of life" happens beneath our feet.

Since the latter half of the 20th century, though, our soil has taken a metaphorical beating, resulting in fake nutrition for the planet. Fake nutrition comes from crops that have been fertilized with a shower of isolated chemical compounds that are supposed to grow plants bigger, better, and faster. What these chemical fertilizers do, however, is pillage the soil by destroying the microbiology and the organic matter within the soil, harming vital nutrients. The blame can be laid at the feet of "Big Ag" and the three synthetically made minerals—nitrogen, phosphorus, and potassium—that have radically changed the nature of farmland dirt in the last fifty to sixty years.

Nitrogen, phosphorus, and potassium—a triumvirate that goes by the acronym NPK—are three of the six primary nutrients or macro-minerals that plants need to sustain continued growth, although there are also dozens of other trace minerals essential to the vitality of plant life.

Nitrogen helps plants make the proteins they need to grow and is a component of chlorophyll, the substance that gives plants their green color. Phosphorous, a key player in the photosynthesis process (the transformation of solar energy into chemical energy), stimulates the root system and helps the plant set buds and flowers. Potassium improves the plant's vigor, promotes blooming, and helps plants resist disease.

In addition to these three main nutrients, plants also need calcium, magnesium, iron, and sulfur as well as micronutrients or trace minerals such as boron, copper, cobalt, and molybdenum to reach their full potential in the plant kingdom.

When these elements are found in rich, dark topsoil, plants experience steady growth and have a far better chance of fighting off pests and disease. When NPK fertilizers are employed, however, plants tend to experience fast, showy growth, which is why they are popular with home gardeners, even though concentrated amounts of NPK fertilizer create the "all show and no go" phenomenon and often "burn" plant life or a backyard lawn. If you've ever tossed too much NPK fertilizer onto a section of grass, then you'll recall how that spot of lawn quickly turned brown and died.

The agriculture industry relies heavily on NPK fertilizers because they tend to plant the same crop on the same land year after year, so farmers feel they have to "goose" their fields by putting back these building blocks of soil into their farmland. What they're doing, however, is applying the same Band-Aid over a wound that grows bigger and bigger with each passing year.

We've now reached the tipping point where the use of NPK fertilizer is ubiquitous and ingrained in the minds of farmers and home gardeners alike. Consider this lead sentence from an article entitled, "Don't Let Your Plants Go Hungry" on the gardeners.com website:

> According to the Gallup Gardening Survey, less than half of the country's home gardeners use any kind of fertilizer on their lawns or gardens. What's unfortunate about this statistic is that it means gardeners aren't getting as many flowers or as much produce as they should. And they're probably struggling with disease and insect problems that could be avoided. Well-fed plants are healthier, more productive, and more beautiful.

Excuse me? "Well-fed" plants are healthier and more productive, even more beautiful than plants and produce grown without NPK fertilizers?

That's a mirage. Come hang out at an organic or biodynamic farm that practices permaculture principles during growing season, and I'll show you vibrant fruits and vegetables that will blow your mind and build your body with real nutrition.

Bottom line: NPK fertilizers do more harm than good. High levels of NPK fertilizers cause the loss of certain plant species, contaminate local drinking water supplies, and prompt the overgrowth of algae in rivers and streams. But their greatest danger is creating an imbalance of nutrients in the soil that causes a depletion of other important minerals such as calcium, copper, and magnesium.

INTRODUCING REAL NUTRITION

Just as there are real and fake nutrients to feed the soil, there are real and fake nutrients in our food. Real nutrition comes from nutrient-dense foods such as kale, red cabbage, spinach, blueberries, strawberries, mangoes, and hundreds of other organically grown fruits, vegetables, seeds, nuts, and legumes as well as sustainably produced animal foods such as wild-caught salmon, pasture-raised organic beef, dairy, and eggs. Real nutrition comes from foods grown in healthy soils that *haven't* been sprayed with NPK fertilizers or pesticides and herbicides.

Real nutrition comes from foods that contain no refined or processed grains, no chemically enhanced oils and fats, and no artificial sweeteners. Real nutrition comes from free-range chickens laying eggs and grass-fed cows, sheep, and goats producing organic meat and dairy products. I've always said that you'll never go wrong eating foods that God created in a form that is healthy for the body.

Just as conventional wisdom says that you need to douse your flowerbeds and garden plots with NPK fertilizer to get the most out of your land, those in the commercial food-producing businesses are constantly researching how they can grow, harvest, transport, process, and mass-produce foods faster and cheaper than the other guy. The major food conglomerates are constantly assessing how they can gain a leg up on the competition. One marketing advantage they like to advertise is that their boxed, bagged, or prepared food has been "fortified" with certain vitamins and minerals.

Commercial bread, even some "wheat" sandwich breads and dinner rolls, is made from enriched wheat flour, which is an oxymoron than ranks right up there with "boneless ribs," "jumbo shrimp," and "natural chemicals."

Wheat flour comes from wheat, of course, and for thousands of years, wheat grain has been a staple of human existence in fresh bread and porridges, and baked bread has been a bulwark against hunger since biblical times. Wheat cultivates easily, stores for years in kernel form, and, when milled into fresh flour, contains beneficial nutrients—although, as we'll discuss later, modern wheat and other gluten-containing grains pose a health risk for many people.

For centuries, the milling process was simple: following the harvest, the wheat grain was ground with a mortar and pestle—a stone club striking grain in a stone bowl—to produce flour. The invention of stone mills powered by water or wind (that's why they have windmills in the Netherlands and waterwheels throughout the rest of Europe) made the labor-intensive process easier. The movement of the stones crushed the entire kernel of grain, which is made up of three parts: the bran, the germ, and the endosperm. Bread produced from these whole grains in ancient times was tremendously healthful.

The advent of the Industrial Revolution changed everything. In the 1870s, the invention of the modern steel roller mill dramatically altered grain milling. Compared to the old stone methods, this new milling method was fast and efficient. Instead of mashing everything together, one could "separate the wheat from the chaff" by breaking up the bran, the germ, and the endosperm at a fraction of the cost of hand-milled wheat.

The cost of wheat flour dropped so dramatically that every class of people in the rapidly growing cities could afford the newfangled "fancy flour." Hailed as a sign of progress, the wide availability and acceptance of modern flour shuttered stone mills in windmills and waterwheels throughout the Western world. White flour became our first processed food and jump-started an industrial food system that led to the production of breads, rolls, crackers, breadsticks, doughnuts, cakes, muffins, and cupcakes in large factories that were shipped to various stores many miles from the point of consumption. Sandwiches—the idea of sticking meat between two pieces of bread—caught on, and the first commercially packaged sliced bread was introduced in 1928, thus giving birth to the saying, "The best thing since sliced bread."

The trouble with the sliced bread was that industrial milling eliminated the bran and germ—the parts of the wheat kernel rich in fiber, proteins, vitamins, lipids, and minerals. This was done to avoid having the flour turn rancid, prevent the development of mold and fungus, and extend the shelf life of the flour and any baked products. To give flour its bright-white color, the wheat stalks were rinsed with various chemical bleaches that sounded like a vocabulary test from high school biology class: nitrogen oxide, chlorine, chloride, nitrosyl, and benzoyl peroxide.

What food manufacturers were doing was taking a healthy food that had been served to families for centuries—usually in the form of bread, pasta, or baked goods—and turning it into one of the most highly allergenic, difficult-to-digest substances on the planet. As I'm fond of saying, the whiter the bread, the sooner you're dead.

The major food manufacturers in the 1930s knew about the loss of essential nutrients, so they began working on ways to produce "enriched flour," which is another oxymoron. Why have a manufacturing process that removes the bran and the germ, which contain fiber and nutrients that the body needs, only to add something back to take their place?

No one was asking that question because the American Medical Association's Council of Foods and Nutrition and the Council on Pharmacy and Chemistry issued a statement in 1938 supporting the fortification of flour and staple foods to combat deficiency-related diseases. At the time, bakers began to voluntarily enrich bread with high-vitamin yeast (which is actually a decent source of nutrients), and by the start of World War II, approximately 75 percent of flour and white bread produced in the U.S. was voluntarily enriched with thiamin, niacin, iron, and dry milk.

Fast forward seventy-five years, and today it's hard to find commercial flour that hasn't been "enriched" with isolated and synthetic vitamins and minerals such as folic acid, riboflavin, niacin, and thiamine. None of those nutrients compare with the quality and potency of the vitamins and minerals found in bran and germ, but the medical establishment and U.S. government's insistence that enriching flour and dairy products dramatically reduces diseases caused by vitamin deficiencies has carried the day.

Everywhere you look on supermarket shelves and dairy cases, you'll find foods and products that are "enriched" and/or "fortified." Examples include vitamin D in milk, fruit juices, and soymilk; folic acid in pastas, rice, and flour; calcium in a variety of dairy products as well as soymilk; and iron (niacin) in breakfast cereals. But enriching foods with synthetic nutrients reminds me of the story about a thief taking your wallet with $100 in cash and handing you a few bucks so you can buy bus fare for the ride home. It's a lopsided deal not in your favor.

Enriching and fortifying our foods is one more example of fake nutrition that started with fertilizing our fields with NPK fertilizers. I prefer to focus on obtaining real nutrition for the planet and the people, which is accomplished by consuming real food produced from rich topsoil that has experienced the short- and long-term breakdown of organic materials. Fake nutrition for the planet and its people is the application and consumption of isolated chemicals that look like nutrients but are made in a laboratory.

Judith DaCava, author of *The Real Truth About Vitamins & Antioxidants*, explains why it's far better to eat whole foods than consuming foods and supplements made from synthetically created vitamins and minerals that were fractionalized by the manufacturing process. Whereas the vitamins, minerals, and enzymes in real foods work together in synergistic fashion, "fortified" foods and nutritional supplements made from synthetic chemical sources react very differently in the body and cause major imbalances.

When you consume whole foods in their natural state, the body is better equipped to "grab" the vitamins and minerals it needs and excrete the rest, while the same nutrients from fortified foods and synthetic supplements cause the body to react as if they were chemicals and even toxic substances, which force the body to react with little opportunity to eliminate the unused material.

So yes, I said it: the synthetic, isolated, chemical vitamins and minerals found in fortified foods and nearly all nutritional supplements *can* be toxic. Examining this statement, one would logically ask: How have we strayed so far in our quest to feed our bodies the nutrients we need?

DO WE NEED TO SUPPLEMENT?

It's easy to think that consuming foods with a wide variety of vitamins and minerals is the end all and be all of living healthy. There's no doubt that vitamins and minerals *are* essential to good health, but I think we can all agree that today's foods lack the nutritional punch they carried more than fifty years ago for reasons that I've described:

soil depletion, the use of fertilizers and pesticides, and the rise of processed and manufactured foods. Is it possible that our quest to obtain vibrant health through the consumption of vitamins and minerals has us barking up the wrong tree?

Many of us try to cover our bases by taking nutritional supplements, which offer a concentrated source of nutrients that today's plant and animal foods don't always provide. In doing so, we may be missing out on real nutrition.

The classic definition for vitamins is that they consist of a group of multifaceted organic substances that regulate metabolism and are required in our daily diets for normal growth and maintenance of life. In reality, though, vitamins are extremely complex substances needed for the human body to work correctly.

The scientific discovery that vitamins and minerals exist isn't that old—just a hundred years or so. Before the 1920s, scientists and learned men and women could only make educated guesses that there had to be *something* microscopic in foods that sustained us. After all, even the most casual observer of the human condition understood that food was a source of energy and sustained life.

Since time immemorial, sick people had called upon medicine men, elders of the tribe, and experienced mothers to "prescribe" certain foods to cure whatever ailed them. Folk medicine helped the ill and the ailing get well, and various healing modalities sprung up organically among people groups across the globe, especially in the Far East and Asia. What may surprise you is the fact that these ancient peoples *did not* focus on vitamins and minerals to attain and regain their health.

Traditional Chinese medicine is perhaps the oldest of all these healing modalities, operating under the belief that the processes of the human body are interrelated and connected to the environment around us. Established thousands of years ago before the birth of Christ, traditional Chinese medicine's central belief is that "life energy," or qi, flows through a number of channels, or meridians, throughout the body by following major veins and arteries and the way they connect to internal organs.

Chinese traditional medicine is also popular in Japan and Taiwan, where it has been adapted to the local culture and is known as **kampo medicine**. Besides employing acupuncture, kampo medicine relies primarily on the prescription of herbal formulas.

Another ancient healing philosophy comes from India, also practiced for thousands of years. Called **Ayurvedic medicine** but also known as **Ayurveda**, this traditional health system emphasizes re-establishing balance in the body through diet, lifestyle, exercise, and body cleansing. Based on the belief that health and wellness depend on a delicate balance between the mind, body, and spirit, the primary focal point of Ayurveda is promoting good health rather than fighting disease.

Closer to home, the healing traditions of many of the indigenous **Native American tribes** learned that by mixing herbs, roots, and other natural plants in their habitat they could heal various medical problems.

The reason I'm bringing up these various traditional medicines is that the tribal elders, medicine men, or learned practitioners never looked upon a sick or weak person and said, "Oh, you're deficient in vitamin C" or "The color of your skin tells me you're not getting enough zinc." Even before vitamins and minerals were discovered, they somehow knew that certain botanicals, herbs, and spices—as well as other natural compounds—had healing properties that could not be denied.

For example, the Ayurvedic medical practitioners of yesteryear weren't concerned with the vitamin and mineral content of the herb known as ashwagandha, but they did know somehow that ashwagandha contained substances beneficial to human health.

Today we call these substances *phytonutrients*. In the case of ashwagandha, modern science has determined that this Indian herb has thirty-four natural phytonutrients ranging from 4-Beta-hydroxywithanolide to withanolide-E. These phytonutrients include antioxidants known to reduce inflammation as well as acting powerfully as a stress reducer.

Turmeric, a bright yellow root native to India and obtained from a plant in the ginger family, has curcuminoids (natural compounds) that are powerful phytonutrients that reduce inflammation, promote brain health, and boost immunity.

Closer to home, Native Americans discovered that pinkish-purple coneflowers called echinacea helped during times they were feeling under the weather with modern studies showing a reduction in time and severity of colds and flus. The tribal elders didn't know about the presence of certain compounds such as alkamides that supported immune response, but that's not my point.

What I'm attempting to draw attention to is that before nutritional supplements were widely available, before vitamins and minerals were discovered, there were phytonutrients in plants and herbs that demonstrated extraordinary health and healing properties. I call them phytonutrient complexes or NewTrients. After nearly twenty years of nutritional research, my contention is that by consuming a diet rich in phytonutrients, or NewTrients, one can truly achieve vibrant health.

So in a *Lion King* sort of way, I'm going to show you how nutritional supplements have come full circle in the last one hundred years.

BACK TO THE FUTURE

I would hope that even the most casual observer of his or her health would agree that the enzymes, minerals, and microorganisms found in today's foods don't measure up to what our ancestors ate many generations ago. Have you tasted a tomato lately?

The idea that our foods lack nutritional zip gained steam right around the time when rapid changes were happening in the way we manufactured and produced food in the 1920s and 1930s. A few health-minded individuals of that time figured out that the new, processed foods showing up in markets were detrimental to good health because they were produced from storehouses of refined white flour and processed sugar.

Out of this development came the idea that we should supplement our diets with the missing nutrients. It was during the Great Depression that we started to see the first "multivitamins" on the market, which were actually dried foods. One such dried food supplement that became very popular was a blend of wheat and barley grasses that could be mixed into your favorite juice or milk. These cereal grasses, as they were known, gained a following rather quickly.

Desiccated liver tablets also became popular, thanks to Charles Atlas—one of the first bodybuilders and fitness buffs to make a name for himself. He promoted taking desiccated liver tablets, a dried or dehydrated form of the organ meat that was reputedly ten to one hundred times higher in nutrients than muscle meat. While nutritional supplements made from dried food closely resembled the foods from which they came, they utilized crude drying methods. When it came to cereal grasses, they were difficult to digest and absorb due to their high fiber content and lack of enzymes.

Once dried food supplements such as wheat grass and desiccated liver made a mark, though, their popularity spurred the development of nutritional supplements made from nutrients that were "extracted" from foods, including various plants such as carrots, acerola cherries, and alfalfa. These provided higher levels of nutrients per serving but were expensive to manufacture.

At the time, in the pre-World War II years, biochemists had discerned that there were thirteen vitamins and divided them into two primary classes according to their solubility in water or fats. Those that dissolved in fat, or were fat-soluble, were vitamins A, D, E, and K. Those that dissolved in water, or were water-soluble, were vitamin C and a group of molecules referred to as the vitamin B complex such as vitamin B_1, B_2, biotin, and folic acid.

Biochemists were learning that vitamin C strengthens tissue such as collagen (this is how vitamin C received its name) gums and muscles, and the body called upon this nutrient to promote healthy skin and support the immune system. They also discovered that vitamin C was mainly found in citrus fruits like rose hips, strawberries, acerola cherries, green and red peppers, tomatoes, broccoli, spinach, and cabbage.

As I mentioned earlier, extracting vitamin C from fruits and vegetables was costly. Biochemists such as Albert Szent-Györgyi of Budapest, Hungary and C.G. King at the University of Pittsburgh were able to extract hexuronic acid—what vitamin C was called in the early days—from citrus fruit and paprika. After Szent-Györgyi put the citrus and paprika through two dozen steps of isolation, purification, and crystallization, he produced a white crystalline powder of even greater purity that he named "ascorbic acid" because it prevented *scorbutus*, the formal Latin name for scurvy.

The scientific community credited Szent-Györgyi for being the first scientist to successfully "isolate" vitamin C in the form of ascorbic acid and awarded him the Nobel Prize in 1937. News of Szent-Györgyi winning science's most prestigious award turned him into an overnight celebrity in Hungary and around the world. A *Time* magazine feature story dated November 1, 1937 said, "In his own backyard, this far-traveling researcher found that paprika was the best source of vitamin C on earth." As winner of the Nobel Prize for Medicine, Szent-Györgyi collected $40,000, worth $600,000 in today's dollars. Despite this ingenious scientist's best efforts, however, ascorbic acid in crystalline form was a far cry from the vitamin C complex contained in the original citrus and paprika.

When the United States went to war in the early 1940s to fight the Axis powers—Germany, Italy, and Japan—research of nutritional supplements was put on the back burner. Following the war, chemical scientists got back to work and discovered many new ways to "isolate" or synthetically replicate nutrients in the laboratory.

Let's take a look at the B vitamins. Vitamin B_1 was the same as thiamine. Vitamin B_2 was isolated as riboflavin, B_6 came out as pyridoxine hydrochloride, and vitamin B_{12} came in as cyanocobalamin.

These synthetic versions dropped the price of vitamin supplements to a level that made them readily affordable to the masses. Manufacturers didn't expect—or desire—that consumers would understand the fine print on the labels affixed to the back of the bottle. For example, if a bottle of chewable vitamin C tablets listed ascorbic acid as its first (and therefore main) ingredient, no one was any the wiser that this compound had been created in a laboratory. If someone picked up a bottle of vitamin E and noticed the main ingredient was dl-alpha tocopheryl, she had no idea she was taking a synthetic version.

As author Judith DaCava pointed out, the body doesn't absorb isolated, synthetic vitamins and minerals very well, which led to the development of the next generation of supplementation—chelated minerals and new forms of vitamins. Chelated minerals were combined chemically with amino acids to form "complexes." For instance, you can purchase chelated calcium or chelated chromium with the idea that these minerals will be better absorbed by the body than isolated, synthetic vitamins and minerals.

Chelated minerals had a good run until fermented nutrients took supplementation to the next level. This was the idea that we needed to go back to multi-complexed nutrients to supplement our diets. Was it possible to develop "whole food" nutrients that came close to food without the bulk of the food?

I gave it a try as I formulated dozens of nutritional supplements that contained ingredients produced by yeast and bacterial fermentation. Fermented vitamins and minerals were made by adding isolated vitamins and minerals into a living yeast or bacterial culture, and with the help of certain amino acids, they created a "whole food" complex. While certainly a step in the right direction, these microorganism/nutrient complexes were essentially the combination of a single-celled organism and an isolated/synthetic nutrient.

In the last few years, I've been seeing extracted or concentrated nutrients in supplements lining health food store shelves. These nutrients, labeled as organic, start with foods and herbs and undergo multiple processing and purification steps without the use of chemical solvents. The organic vitamin and mineral supplements available today are well formulated and devoid of chemicals, but they are highly purified and processed, which makes them a far cry from the food from which they came.

After nearly twenty years of research on human nutrition, I believe if I had to choose one of the previous vitamin/mineral iterations, I'd have to go with the dried food supplements of old. But in my recent nutritional developments, I've stumbled upon a few age-old secrets that I believe will change the way we supplement our diets forever.

To complete the nutritional supplement "circle of life," while paying homage to the ancients, I have felt compelled to go back to the nutritional drawing board and develop a real-food supplement solution to provide key phytonutrients, or NewTrients, in a form that the body can truly use while respecting the environment from which the food came.

When I talk about real nutrition supplements, I believe in the utilization of ancient, artisanal techniques. In the last two years, I've been researching and developing what I believe will be the next great movement in nutritional supplementation—the real food movement. I believe, as the ancients have taught us, that food truly nourishes our bodies. The closer our supplements are to real-foods, the closer we will be to vibrant health.

Before I reveal this amazing nutritional discovery, I think it's important to lay out a dietary roadmap that can benefit everyone reading these words. The main theme of *Planet Heal Thyself* is revealed in ten principles outlined in the following chapters. In addition to consuming real nutrition, you will learn how to unlock and even transform the nutrients found in the most healthful foods and how you can incorporate them into your daily diet.

By following the principles I call the Get Real 10, you can begin a transformation in body, mind, and planet.

For more information on Real Food Nutrients, I invite you to visit www.PlanetHealThyself.com.

2

Sprouting to Life

I'M A HUGE FAN OF SPROUTED FOODS, SO ONE THING WE'VE DONE AT the Heal the Planet Farm is purchase our own commercial sprouter. It's a luxury, for sure, but you should see our sprouting system that automatically washes, sanitizes, rinses, soaks, germinates, and grows various seeds in a continuous flow. The sprouter mists the seeds all day and all night long, providing them the continual stimulus they need to explode with nutrition.

I love walking over to our small restaurant-style kitchen in the morning and reaching in for a handful of sprouted broccoli seeds or seeds from sprouted clover, sprouted rye grass, or even sprouted onion. The seeds can be fairly fibrous, so chewing on a mouthful can take a while—kind of like chewing gum. I don't mind because chomping on sprouted seeds means I'm consuming a live food brimming with vitamins, minerals, enzymes, and phytonutrients. Eating sprouted seeds packs quite a nutritional wallop and punch well beyond their weight.

By definition, sprouts are edible plant seeds that are germinated—meaning they're beginning to grow and show their first edible shoots. Like other vegetable foods, sprouts can vary in texture and taste. Perhaps you're acquainted with hardy bean sprouts (small, light yellow leaves and silvery white shoots) or threadlike alfalfa sprouts (thin, delicate, and green), which are readily available at your local supermarket or health food store.

My favorite at the farm are the sprouted broccoli seeds, which are much more potent than this Italian heirloom vegetable brought to America in the 1880s. I can't say I totally enjoy the radish-like taste of broccoli seeds, but they're a superstar sprout because of the way they act as an antioxidant to stimulate the cells' ability to protect our body from immune system onslaught.

Sprouted broccoli seeds have been the subject of major research at Johns Hopkins University over the years. In the late 1990s, research teams at Johns Hopkins released studies concluding that broccoli sprouts contained thirty to fifty times the concentration of powerful antioxidant compounds than the familiar broccoli florets that often decorate dinner plates. A high concentration of protective chemicals, called isothiocyanates, make broccoli seeds potent stimulators of natural detoxifying enzymes in the body. And in 2014, Johns Hopkins announced the results of a clinical trial suggesting that broccoli sprouts may improve behavior in struggling children.

I've been consuming sprouted seeds for a long time. I love how sprouts are growing at the same moment you're harvesting and consuming them—meaning you're capturing live nutrients at their nutritional peak. It's my view, though, that not nearly enough of us are intentional about including sprouted foods in our diets. We'll regularly eat lettuce-and-tomato salads until the cows come home, but including a dollop of sprouts is an afterthought for many. Furthermore, sprouting seeds at home, while a great concept, is not on many people's radar screens.

That's why I hope to inspire you to think about including more sprouted foods in your diet. When it comes to the revolution of regeneration, the second principle of the Get Real 10—*eat sprouted food*—is a great way to raise the health of your body as well as our planet.

THE HEALTH BENEFITS OF SPROUTING

Sprouting is the practice of soaking seeds overnight, then repeatedly rinsing them until they develop tail-like protrusions that keep on growing. In addition to veggies, you can successfully sprout nuts, grains, legumes, and beans as well. And just so you know, I'm a big believer in the benefits of consuming sprouted grains in breads, pastas, and cereals over their non-germinated counterparts. I don't eat much bread these days, but when I do, sprouted bread has been a favorite for nearly twenty years. I prefer to consume sprouted gluten-free grains for reasons I'll share in an upcoming chapter.

The reason I recommend eating sprouted food is because the soaking process turns these seeds into tiny nutritional powerhouses with readily bioavailable vitamins, minerals, and proteins plus beneficial enzymes and phytochemicals. Sprouting also breaks down the natural agents—known as anti-nutrients—in the seed's outer coating that protect the seeds from early germination and predators. One of these anti-nutrients is phytic acid, which can do a number on your digestive system.

If you've had difficulties digesting seeds, sprouting will help a great deal because phytic acid, which also blocks the absorption of calcium and magnesium, is largely decomposed by the soaking process. Soaking and germination also breaks down complex sugars responsible for causing intestinal gas while neutralizing enzyme inhibitors and activating beneficial enzymes that break down other indigestible toxins.

Dr. Edward Howell, one of my nutritional heroes and author of *Enzymes for Health and Longevity*, wrote that germination increases the enzyme activity by as much as six times. This is due to proteolytic release of the enzymes by inactivation of the enzyme inhibitors found in all seeds. What this means in simpler English is that soaking and sprouting breaks down the seed into its simplest components, such as proteins into amino acids and complex starches into simpler carbohydrates or sugars, which intensifies the nutrient content. Sprouting allows proteases within to neutralize any inhibiting factors and release the enzymes from bondage.

Sprouting unlocks food's goodness in many ways. Sally Fallon, co-author of *Nourishing Traditions*, said that the process of germination not only produces vitamin C, but also changes the composition of seeds in numerous beneficial ways. Sprouting increases vitamin B content, especially B_2, B_5 and B_6. Carotene increases dramatically—sometimes eightfold. Even more important, sprouting neutralizes enzyme inhibitors present in all seeds.

How do you sprout your own seeds?

Few can justify a commercial sprouter like the one we own at the Heal the Planet Farm, but there are several DIY approaches you can take. The simplest and least inexpensive route is purchasing:

- a quart-sized canning jar
- a wide-mouth canning ring
- a sprouting screen
- sprouting seeds (broccoli, clover, or whatever fits your fancy)

The first thing you need to do is soak your sprouting seeds overnight. After dinner, pour about 3 tablespoons of your sprouting seeds into the bottom of your quart jar. Put your sprouting screen in place at the top of the quart jar and screw on the canning ring. Pour about two cups of filtered, non-chlorinated water through the sprout screen. Swirl the water around the seeds, drain the water, and pour another two to four cups of water on the seeds. Then leave your jar on your kitchen countertop. That's all you need to do the first night.

In the morning, you can drain the water out. Then you want to repeat the process of rinsing, swirling, and draining. When you feel the jar has been drained well, place it in a small bowl that will allow the jar to lay at a slight angle, pointing down, which will allow any excess water to drain out. Continue rinsing and draining throughout the first day, probably two or three times.

Over the next several days, you'll start to see the first shoots of sprouts grow and fill the quart jar. After five or six days, your sprouted seeds should be ready to eat or stored in the refrigerator for consumption later. If kept dry, the sprouts will last several days. You can eat them out of your hand, like I do, mix them into your salad, or pile them onto your sandwiches.

You can find starter kits online that will help newbies with printed instructions and various sets of seeds to use with a growing container. If you're going to give sprouting at home a shot, I recommend that you start with vegetable seeds such as broccoli, alfalfa, or clover like we've done at the Heal the Planet Farm.

LOOKING TO THE PLANET

Sprouting happens in nature through a process called germination, or the way the planet allows food to come forth from the soil. Because of a symbiotic relationship, nature transforms topsoil and therefore its produce in one of three ways:

1. fermentation

2. sprouting

3. super-heating

Let me describe what this trio of items means to the planet. **Fermentation** refers to enriching the soil to maximize plant productivity. I've already discussed how the soils of our planet are comprised of natural microorganisms that—when balanced— harmonize in a natural fermentative environment. Composting organic matter regenerates the soil and slowly feeds the planet in a time-release fashion.

The **sprouting** or germination process helps to build soil organic matter, protecting and regenerating the planet, in one of two ways: through shading the Earth from the intense rays of the sun and erosion-causing wind, or from the sprout growing and creating an abundant food source for animals who consume the plant and return a significant portion of the nutrition back into the soil in the form of excrement (manure).

When healthy sprouted plant material covers the ground, it's protecting topsoil from scorching and wind erosion while helping the planet retain what it needs—moisture and nutrients. I've walked out onto fields at our Heal the Planet Farm in the middle of a blazing hot summer day, well into the 90s, but if I put my hand under a canopy of red clover and orchard grass, the temperature of the soil could be 10 to 15 degrees cooler. I can also feel moisture in the soil, which is incredible to me.

Even better is when sprouted plant material feeds grazing cattle, sheep, and goats. These animals, in turn, recycle anywhere from 60 percent to 80 percent of these nutrients when they leave behind their urine and manure. The circle of life is completed when these animals die and their decaying bodies fertilize the soil, adding beneficial macro- and micronutrients.

Grazing animals get a bad rap in some environmental circles, but I believe they can play a pivotal role in healing the planet. For example, if you have a corn field that you plant and decide not to harvest but allow the corn to sprout, ripen, and eventually fall to the ground, it will take a long time for the stalks and fallen corn cobs to break down and feed the soil. But if cattle, sheep, or goats come in and eat the green grass around the stalks, trample what they don't eat, *and* litter the area with urine and manure, the "pre-digested" nutrients in their manure and nitrogen in the urine provide readily available fertility to the soil.

At the Heal the Planet Farm, we've designed a mixed species, high-pressure, rotational grazing system so that our animals can consume large amounts of forage in short amounts of time while effectively fertilizing the ground by evenly distributing their urine and manure and trampling the little they don't eat. At most dairy farms and cattle ranches around the country, though, the animals are spread out on a large field for long periods of time, providing little grazing pressure and where there will either be one pond or one well for the animals to hydrate themselves.

What happens in this scenario is that the manure tends to pile up around the watering hole or along the trail to the pond without being evenly spread throughout the land. What we've done at our farm to counteract this trend is to set out small "paddocks," following a strategic grazing pattern with high pressure and rapid livestock moves in a mixed species grazing system, allowing for thorough fertilization and rapid soil building. By planting seed immediately before or after each paddock is grazed, the ability to build soil organic matter and create an increase in plant biomass with each grazing season becomes a reality.

As for the **super-heating** process, I'm referring to the accelerated breakdown and release of carbon through subjecting organic material to high temperatures. In nature, this is accomplished through the use of fire, which can be an important management tool for maintaining and enhancing grasslands. There have been times when I've been driving around my Missouri farmlands on an all-terrain vehicle and come upon a grazing field that's a deeper emerald green than the rest.

"How come that field is so green?" I'll ask one of the farmhands.

"Oh, that's where a brush fire broke out last fall," he'll reply.

Around the Heal the Planet Farm, we have a handful of "burned fields" that are a more vibrant green during the growing season. Some of our fields burned from lightning strikes, but sometimes a neighbor will burn his field intentionally—known as a prescribed burn—and the fire "jumps" the property line.

Whether an act of nature or purposely set, fire rejuvenates open areas to create lush and healthy grasslands by "cleansing" the topsoil and stimulating plant growth. Even though I don't like the idea of releasing that much carbon into the atmosphere when a field burns, this mode of super-heating is a far more acceptable way for the planet to heal itself than by invasive plowing to clear out old growth and start anew.

MAKING A STEP TOWARD SPROUTED FOODS

I believe I've successfully built a case that sprouting increases favorable compounds in foods and that nutrient and enzyme levels are greatly increased as a result of germination. As a double benefit, the negative anti-nutrients you find in seeds, legumes, and grains are greatly reduced.

Sprouts are a superfood that many tend to overlook, and I think I know why. It's because it takes effort to seek out seeds suitable for sprouting and then looking after the "wash and rinse" cycle for several days. Even if that's the case for you, let me leave you with a few closing thoughts about sprouts:

Sprouts have a nutritional profile that's amazing.

Sprouts have high levels of dietary fiber, B complex vitamins, protein, digestive enzymes, and some of the highest known levels of powerful antioxidants. It's all due to the initiation of the seed-soaking process, which eliminates harmful compounds, and their germination causes nutrients to explode within the seed.

Sprouts are about as "live" a food as you can find.

Even the healthiest vegetables lose a significant percentage of their nutrients in their trip from farm to table. You could say that sprouted seeds are still "growing" until the moment you take a bite.

Sprouts supply food in a pre-digested form.

In other words, sprouted food has an abundance of enzymes, which makes them easy to digest. Sprouting also breaks down enzyme and nutrient inhibitors, which allows your body to readily absorb calcium, magnesium, iron, copper, and zinc.

Sprouts give you a great bang for your shopping dollar.

Everyone knows that organic vegetables don't come cheap these days, but sprouts can be inexpensive, especially when you're making your own.

Sprouts are a complete food source and biologically efficient.

There is a plethora of live vitamins, minerals, proteins, enzymes, and even chlorophyll in every handful of sprouts.

You can grow sprouts year-round, even in cold-weather climates.

In the nation's snow belts, it's difficult to find fresh vegetables in the middle of winter. (And those green foods spent days sitting inside a refrigerated truck to reach your local supermarket or health food store.) But with a sprouting kit, sprouts come to life in your kitchen any time you want and don't take up any space at all.

Sprouts make a great ingredient in any sandwich.

Kids—and adults—love sandwiches, so instead of using green lettuce or watery tomatoes, include sprouts as you make your sandwiches. Sprouts have a way of tasting great with sprouted whole grain bread.

Sprouts can help you lose weight.

Let's say you go crazy and add a whole cup of alfalfa sprouts to your salad. If so, you've only added eight calories to your meal and provided nutrients and fiber to curb your appetite. In a way, consuming sprouts is anti-caloric, meaning that it takes more energy to digest the sprouts than they provide in the form of calories.

Whether you decide to start sprouting on your own or shop for items such as alfalfa sprouts, mung bean sprouts, or broccoli seeds, consuming sprouted foods is a great way to start healing your body as well as the planet. Eating sprouted seeds means you're consuming a live food at the peak of its nutritional value.

For those of you who consume dietary supplements, there is a new generation of real-food nutritional products that utilize organic sprouted ingredients, which I believe to be a breakthrough in health and wellness. When shopping at your local health food store, look for foods and supplements made with sprouted ingredients.

In my next chapter, I'll talk about fermentation and how this ancient wisdom combined with modern technology can help transform our bodies and heal our planet.

For more information on incorporating sprouted foods into your daily diet, visit www.PlanetHealThyself.com.

3

Fantastic Fermentation

I WAS FIRST EXPOSED TO A "REGENERATIVE/SUSTAINABLE LIFESTYLE" when I was a young boy, even though I didn't know it at the time and the phrase hadn't been coined yet.

It all happened because of my grandfather, Papa Jerry. I can remember, when I was five or six years old, visiting him and Grandma Ann at their single-family row house on Long Island, outside of New York City. My grandparents had a small back yard that was all garden and no lawn.

Papa Jerry, who had a great passion for gardening, ripped out his green grass to cultivate a vegetable plot, using every available square inch to plant cucumbers, tomatoes, and lettuce. Peach and pear trees delivered delicious fresh fruit.

The deep, dark soil was incredibly fertile because of a compost pile that took up a big corner of the yard. I can remember Papa Jerry leading me over to the large mound of dirt, proud as can be. "Just put your hands in the soil, Jordi, and let it slide over your hands. Don't you feel the richness and life in that dirt? The black color means the soil is rich in nutrients."

As a first-grader, the only thing that impressed me was sticking a shovel into the compost pile and disturbing hundreds of squirming earthworms. My grandfather was an avid composter who made sure that every bit of garbage and food scraps made it onto his beloved pile of dirt. He even got a bucket brigade going when I took a bath, insisting that we dump the dirty bathwater on top of the compost. "That's why we have the largest red tomatoes in the neighborhood," Papa Jerry said with a tinge of pride.

Growing up in the South Florida suburbs during my adolescent years, amid the swaying palm trees and blue-green dense turf comprised of St. Augustine grass, didn't give me much opportunity to get my hands dirty after Papa Jerry died from a sudden heart attack when I was nine years old. I didn't know it at the time, but my next firsthand experience with composting wouldn't happen for more than twenty-five years when we purchased our own farmland.

Thanks to Papa Jerry, I knew something about composting when we started our Heal the Planet Farm, which was a good thing because I had to come up to speed quickly after learning our topsoil was in trouble. Trucking in organic topsoil—an expensive proposition—wasn't an option, but rebuilding our soil through composting could restore the health of our farmland slowly but surely.

I mentioned in the Introduction how one of our key soil-building programs combines manure waste from our organic dairy operation with untreated oak wood chips and our leftover food and kitchen garbage to create one of the best composting operations east of the Hudson River. Whenever the kids dump a pail filled with a grimy mix of banana peels, cheese rinds, onion scraps, eggshells, and watermelon rinds on top of the pile, our chickens go to town. They peck and poop all day long, leaving deposits of chicken litter everywhere they go. Their poultry poop has some of the highest nitrogen levels of any domesticated animal's manure and is known for helping turn compost into "black gold."

It's been interesting to see what the chickens love getting their beaks into. To our surprise, chickens *love* watermelon rinds and will peck at the white rinds until the smooth, green outer skin rolls up like gift-wrap paper. Our chickens also have sophisticated palates because they go crazy over cheese and red onions.

I never thought I could get so excited about chickens, manure, and compost, but the point I want to get across is that composting is nature's way of using fermentation to transform difficult-to-digest food scraps and compounds into useable materials for rebuilding the soil. That's a good thing because food scraps make up 20 percent to 30 percent of what we throw away and are the largest category of municipal solid waste hauled away to the nearest landfill, according to the U.S. Environmental Protection Agency.

In 2012, the most recent year for which estimates are available, Americans tossed more than 35 million tons of food waste into their garbage cans and dumpsters. Or, said another way, we throw out more food than all the plastic, paper, metal, and glass combined—which means a lot of food spoils or never gets eaten. Unfortunately, only 4 percent of our food waste is diverted from landfills and incinerators for composting.

Composting food scraps and other waste products is one of the best ways you can help the planet heal itself. Keeping these materials out of landfills and producing rich compost can help houseplants grow, improve vegetable gardens, and make lawns greener. Composting is a win-win for the environment and your wallet.

I have a great feeling every time one of the kids carries the slop bucket out to our composting pile, where the chickens can get started on breakfast, lunch, and dinner and do their part to fertilize the soil beneath their orange claws. I feel good knowing every bit of leftover organic food and kitchen waste ends up turning into rich soil to cover the earth. Our composting program at the Heal the Planet Farm has made such an impression on me that when I'm on the road, I feel guilty throwing away banana peels, eggshells, or apple cores.

Our family spent the winter of 2014-15 in Central California, not far from San Luis Obispo, where we were able to continue composting at our rental property. One thing I learned while wintering in California is that composting is catching on in the Golden State, both in agriculture and in the suburbs.

That's great news because decades of over-farming have denuded the vitality of the Central Valley's growing soil. The worry among those in the know is that California's productive agricultural areas—our primary source for tomatoes, almonds, grapes, strawberries, raspberries, salad greens, olives, apricots, and asparagus—are at risk because of the abuse. The deteriorating topsoil took another blow from a severe drought that has gripped California in recent years. The West Coast's last good season of rainfall was in 2010-11, so the devastating drought has exacerbated a dire situation. If the drought continues, the Central Valley might face the same devastation as the Midwestern Dust Bowl of the 1930s.

The ray of sunshine is that a growing number of farmers finally understand that their farmlands and their livelihoods are on the line if something isn't done to enrich their topsoil. I have a friend in organic farming in the Central Valley who buys compost by the truckload from companies like Kochergen Farms Composting, certified in producing organic compost. Companies like Kochergen receive the postproduction pulp and rinds from orange juice manufacturers, lettuce and cabbage from producers who trim, peel, and cut off leaves, grape skins and stems from winemakers, or any fruit and vegetables leftovers they can get their hands on to make composted soil.

Statewide, big cities are getting behind composting. The City of Los Angeles has been hauling dozens of eighteen-wheel trucks each day—filled with rotting fruits and vegetables from supermarkets, lawn clippings, and sewage sludge—to the Community Recycling and Resource Recovery's composting facility near Fresno. Other metro areas are getting on board because of a 2011 California state law that mandates that cities and counties must either recycle or reduce 75 percent of its waste by 2020. That's only a few years away.

In 2014, thirty-nine of the Golden State's fifty-eight counties shipped more than 5 percent of their trash and recycling materials to huge composting facilities in the rural Central Valley. That's a great start, but there's plenty of room for sending a lot more food scraps and green waste to compost facilities, where the raw materials are dumped into huge piles that eventually feed and stimulate microorganisms to break down the various foodstuffs.

Recycling is and has been a great way to heal the planet. Perhaps your municipal garbage service is like what I saw in some California locales, where recycling has gotten a lot easier and more user-friendly. Many California households must "separate" their trash into green bins (for leaves, yard clippings, mowed grass, and pulled-up weeds), blue bins (for newspaper and papers, glass containers, aluminum, and plastic jars and containers), and gray bins (for household garbage and food waste).

Finally, there's one other way to compost that I should mention. Composting toilets are an alternative to flush toilets when there are no hookups available to a municipal treatment plant or a septic tank.

I actually have some experience with a composting toilet. My wife, Nicki, and I were presented with a composting toilet just outside our tent when we celebrated our tenth wedding anniversary at the remote Clayoquot Wilderness Retreat off of Vancouver Island in British Columbia. Using a composting toilet took some getting used to, but I guess the experience wasn't all bad because we plan to build and set up composting toilets for employees and visitors at the Heal the Planet Farm.

While composting toilets are great and wonderful for the planet, their widespread usage isn't exactly realistic today. But composting household leftovers, garbage, and even dirty bathwater, like my Papa Jerry did in his back yard, can take your environmental game up a big notch.

COMPOSTING AT HOME

The great news about composting is that you can compost just about anywhere. It doesn't matter where you live. Even apartment and condo dwellers can compost without a backyard or balcony. All you need is a compost bin with a pair of lids, some old newspaper, food scraps, water, and a handful of worms (optional)—preferably red wigglers, the worms of choice for composting.

For indoor use, a compost container can be plastic or ceramic. (Wooden compost bins belong outside the house.) The second lid goes under the container to capture water drainage. The first thing you want to do is shred newspaper or any printouts and then soak the paper in water. Next, fill the container with half of your shredded and soaked paper until it's filled about a third of the way. Add some worms, a bit of soil, and let the container sit in the sunlight. The worms will begin burrowing into the paper.

If you are composting indoors, bring your composting container into the kitchen, where you can store it under the sink, or some place out of way, like a back porch, balcony, laundry room, or garage. (When done correctly, composting containers don't smell or draw pests.) Add food scraps, burying them under your remaining paper scraps, and continue to toss in more scraps (see the list below) until everything's well on the road to being fully composted.

You'd be surprised at all the materials that can be thrown into your compost container. Here's a long but not complete list:

- cardboard rolls from paper towels and toilet paper

- clean paper or newspaper, preferably shredded or torn up

- coffee grounds and filters

- table scraps, including corncobs

- rotting fruits and vegetables

- eggshells (if you have chickens, be sure to break them up so your chickens don't start pecking their own eggs)

- fireplace ashes

- grass clippings

- hair and fur

- cotton rags

- dryer lint

- hay and straw

- houseplants

- shrub prunings

- fall leaves

- peanut shells

- tea bags

- wood chips

- wool rags

And it all turns into rich topsoil. Astonishing what those earthworms can do, right? But some things you *don't* want to put in your indoor compost container are dairy products (yogurt, milk, and cottage cheese), meat scraps, fish bones, grease, and leftover oils because that will create odor problems and attract flies. Pet manure is another no-no. While the aforementioned items are compostable, they are best incorporated into an outdoor composting operation.

Keep your compost moist by watering occasionally as well as covered because this helps retain moisture and heat, two big essentials for composting. When the soil is dark and rich as can be, scoop out the compost (but not the worms) and start all over again. You can use the composted material with potted houseplants or as vegetation around your apartment, condo, or home. You can sprinkle on your lawn or even use as gifts to friends with green thumbs. Dirt—the gift that keeps on giving!

Composting has picked up enough momentum that there's even a *Composting for Dummies* book with the familiar yellow and black cover. Composting is moving into the mainstream, like the story I heard from a California friend who ordered a sandwich at a deli in the wine country. At the last second, he changed his mind on the type of bread he wanted, but the person behind the counter was halfway done making his sandwich.

"Oh, that's no problem," the sandwich maker said, fetching a new whole grain roll. "We'll throw the other bread into our compost pile. It's all good."

A year or two ago, that bread would have been headed for a landfill. Instead, that unused roll will be used to build topsoil and help heal the planet.

Think about giving composting a try. There are tons of resources online to learn more about this practice, but a good first step is to talk to those who compost. Ask questions. Get their take. Touch the fertile topsoil they make.

If you don't know anyone who's into composting, then drop by a farmers market on a Saturday morning. Most likely, nearly every vendor composts because they're likely to be environmentally minded and have to do something with the leftover fruits and vegetables that spoil or don't sell. These are the types of folks who can steer you in the right direction.

THE JOY OF FERMENTED FOODS

Composting is nature's fermentation used to heal the planet, and consuming fermented foods may be the best tool to heal your body.

Fermentation doesn't get talked about a lot around the kitchen table or the conference room because most people aren't really aware of what fermented foods are or that they should be eating them. Yogurt is hardly ever referred to as "fermented milk," and sauerkraut is virtually never called "fermented vegetables," yet that's what they and hundreds of other fantastic, healthful fermented foods can be called. Fermented foods' distinguishing characteristic is that they have a sour, tangy taste that's health giving and can be very pleasurable to eat, at least to me.

So what is fermentation?

Fermentation is the culturing or natural souring of various foods with the intentional growth of bacteria, yeast, fungi, or mold. It's a time-honored method that allows foods to stay edible longer. Without fermentation, you have to wonder if we'd be here—our ancestors could have starved during a long winter if they had to rely on foods they gathered during the harvest season with no way to preserve them. For most of recorded history, fruits, vegetables, dairy, and meats had no "shelf life" unless you put them through a fermentation process.

I suppose our forbearers could have survived a frozen winter on fresh milk from stall-fed cows, goats, or sheep consuming stored grains or by consuming the grains themselves and using them to bake bread, but that would have been thin gruel as they say. Instead, our ancestors learned they could preserve *and* produce excellent, nutritional foods through the process of fermentation.

We don't know how and when the art of fermenting foods began, but we do know from ancient texts, including the Bible, that early people discovered a way to preserve foods from the beginning of time. One of the first actions taken by Noah, following the Great Flood, was to plant a vineyard so that wine could be made.

Abraham entertained three celestial beings with servings of bread, honey, and "curds," which is what we would call cheese today but could mean a thick food reminiscent of strained or green yogurt. A rich landowner named Boaz invited Ruth, who later became his wife, to dip bread into his oil and vinegar.

Fermented foods played a big role in ancient cultures as well. Greek mythology described Dionysus as the god of wine. The Greek philosopher Aristotle praised the healing effects of cured cucumbers, or what is known today as pickles. Roman emperors, including Julius Caesar, fed pickles to their troops in the belief they provided physical and spiritual strength.

Further east, the Chinese started fermenting cabbage before the Common Era, even though it's the Romans who are generally believed to have produced the first sauerkraut. Asians became skilled at preparing elaborate fermented foods such as kimchi, a condiment made up of cabbage, other vegetables, and seasonings. Eastern Europeans discovered ways to pickle green tomatoes, peppers, and lettuce. And in nearly every culture, dairy products have been used to make fermented foods such as yogurt, kefir, cheese, cottage cheese, and cultured cream (also known as crème fraîche or Crème Bulgare).

My Grandma Rose made créme fraîche in an Old Country sort of way. She grew up on a Polish farm in the 1920s, the youngest of seven children in a poor family. The family bartered eggs for milk from the village dairyman, and it fell on Rose's young shoulders to deliver the eggs and lug a tin pail of fresh cow's milk back to the family cellar. This was raw, unpasteurized, and unhomogenized milk—the real deal—and did not have to be refrigerated. Their milk couldn't be refrigerated anyway because "ice boxes," as they were known in those days, were luxury items for city dwellers.

After two or three days in the cellar (one day in warm weather or two to three days in cooler weather), the raw milk would culture and thicken, and Rose and her siblings fought over who would get to taste the tangy cream that formed at the top of the pail. If you've ever enjoyed crème fraîche, then you know what I'm talking about.

What remained in the pail was a type of fermented dairy called "clabbered cream." The explanation for the culturing process is that the bacteria in the milk began the process of converting lactose—milk sugar, so therefore sweet—into lactic acid, which, being an acid, is tart or sour. In addition to changing the taste, this fermentation caused a slight curdling, which thickened the milk as it rose toward the top and turned into a delicious cream.

Fermented foods have been used for centuries for their health-promoting effects. I strongly recommend that you look for ways to consume cultured and fermented dairy products, sauerkraut, real pickles, and Asian-centric miso, tempeh, natto, soy sauce, and kimchi. These are all foods I consume, as well as an amazing African-inspired fermented dairy beverage that I helped re-create in the U.S. It's called Amasai, which has the consistency of a liquid yogurt and provides the body with high-quality proteins, vitamins, minerals, enzymes, probiotics, and healthy fats. The inspiration for Amasai came from *amasi* or *maas*, the traditional dairy beverage of the Maasai tribe.

What history and world cultures have long recorded and known about fermentation is becoming increasingly studied, tested, and accepted in the world of science. We know that fermentation:

- renders food resistant to microbial spoilage and the development of toxins

- inhibits the transfer of pathogenic organisms

- improves digestion and nutrient absorption of food

- preserves food between the time of harvest and consumption

- enhances flavor and nutritional value of food

Preservation of vegetables and fruits by the process of fermentation has numerous advantages beyond those of simple preservation. Starches, sugars, and proteins in vegetables and fruits are converted into organic acids—such as acetic and lactic acid—by the many species of bacteria, yeast, and fungi. These microbes are present on the surface of all living things on this planet and are especially numerous on leaves, roots, and plants growing in or near the ground. In addition to preservation, fermentation induces the transformation of normal foods into super-foods, making them more nutritious and easier to digest and assimilate.

In fact, you could call these microbes "agents of transformation."

TOP SECRET AGENTS

Lactobacilli are but one example of fermentative microorganisms found in cultured foods and beverages. In the rest of this chapter, I'm going to talk about six of these "agents of transformation," which are listed here:

- *Lactobacillus plantarum*

- *Ophiocordyceps (cordyceps) sinensis*

- *Trametes versicolor*

- *Ganoderma lucidum*

- *Hericium erinaceus*

- *Bacillus subtilis*

Don't let the long, tongue-twisting Latin names, based in science, stop you from reading more. These "super six" cultures can go a long way toward improving your health and the environment. Here's a closer look:

1. *Lactobacillus plantarum*

This lactic acid-producing bacterium is commonly found in fermented vegetables. Sauerkraut, pickles, olives, and Korean kimchi are examples. This microorganism found in those foods helps ensure that vitamins and minerals reach your cells.

Scientists call the process of preserving vegetables for a long period of time a form of "lacto-fermentation," which might lead you to believe that dairy products are involved. That's not really the case. Here's what author Sally Fallon had to say in her book, *Nourishing Traditions*:

> Lactic acid is a natural preservative that inhibits putrefying bacteria. Starches and sugars in vegetables and fruits are converted into lactic acid by the many species of lactic acid-producing bacteria. These *lactobacilli* are ubiquitous, present on the surface of living things and especially numerous on leaves and roots of plants growing in or near the ground.... The proliferation of *lactobacilli* in fermented vegetables enhances their digestibility and increases vitamin levels. These beneficial organisms produce numerous helpful enzymes as well as antibiotic and anti-carcinogenic substances. Their main byproduct, lactic acid, not only keeps vegetables and fruits in a state of perfect preservation but also promotes the growth of healthy flora throughout the intestine.

When I first read Sally Fallon's book, *Nourishing Traditions*, in the late 1990s, she made a convincing argument that cultured vegetables could improve gut health, which piqued my interest for more information. My search led me to *The Complete Guide to Raw Cultured Vegetables* by Evan Richards, who made the case that raw cultured vegetables were a rejuvenating source of non-dairy *lactobacilli* such as *Lactobacillus plantarum*.

Today, you could call me a fermentation junkie. I can't eat enough organic sauerkraut, but you want to stay away from the commercial sauerkraut found in the supermarket because it's generally pasteurized—a heating process that destroys the good bacteria as well as the bad—and packed with distilled vinegar and preservatives such as sodium benzoate.

I understand that you may turn up your nose at sauerkraut. *Sorry, Jordan, but I can't stand the taste.* I hear you, but sauerkraut's a taste that can grow on you. Give it a try, perhaps a bit at a time.

Here's a story that might encourage you. One of our children, Isabella, recently came into our care, on the way to an eventual adoption, when she was two years old. When she first arrived, we took her food shopping, and I'll never forget how she pointed out every junk food in the store. Pizza. Ice cream. Candy. Cookies. Chips. She didn't mention any fruits or vegetables she liked…especially vegetables.

Nicki and I patiently explained to her that those weren't healthy foods to eat, which our two-year-old didn't understand, of course. Nonetheless, we stayed the course and fed her what everyone else in the family ate—healthful, organic foods.

Slowly but surely, we got her to try a wonderful array of fruits and vegetables, and yes, even sauerkraut. Fast-forward five months, and we were in the grocery store again. I was pushing her in our shopping cart toward the cooler where the fermented foods were displayed when she immediately took her right fist and pumped it across her body. "Look, Dad! Sauerkraut! I love sauerkraut!"

What we did was help a child move from the cultural tastes for sweet and salty to one that included sour, which is the predominant and beneficial taste that fermentation and bacteria such as *Lactobacillus plantarum* bring to the table.

My daughter now likes my other fermented favorites such as real pickles and a raw combination of red cabbage, beets, carrots, and garlic. These fresh, raw vegetables are ground up, put into a stainless steel container, and left to culture for five to seven days. Because the cultured veggie blend is not pasteurized, the healthy lactobacilli and enzymes contain amazing health benefits.

There have been times when I've had boxes of raw sauerkraut shipped to me, but often the long journey takes its toll on my fermented foods. I can remember opening a box and getting smacked with a sulfur-like smell that filled the entire house. What happened is that a bottle or two of the cultured veggies broke during shipment, but the raw veggies continued to ferment. Phew! Or should I say, whew!

2. *Ophiocordyceps sinensis*

Here's an "agent of transformation" that needs a pronunciation guide: *oh-fee-oh-cord-yee-ceps see-nen-sis*. Never heard of this fungus that attaches itself to ghost moth caterpillars? You would if you lived in rural Tibet, where caterpillars infected with this fungus have sparked a modern-day gold rush—each is worth twice its weight in the precious metal.

In fact, this fungus contributes as much as 80 percent of local villagers' annual income and 8 percent of Tibet's gross national product (GNP), all because of a feverish demand for the naturally occurring "caterpillar fungus" that's prized in China for its health benefits as well as its purported ability to act as an aphrodisiac. The demand is so high that the rare Asian fungus sells for up to $50,000 a pound.

Ophiocordyceps sinensis is the scientific name for the Tibetan term *yartsa gunbu*, a fungus that invades the bodies of ground-burrowing ghost moth caterpillars high up in the Himalayan mountains—past 10,000 feet in elevation. *Ophiocordyceps sinensis* became famous in the U.S. based on its use by the Chinese women athletes in the early 1990s when Wang Junxia ran 10,000 meters 42 seconds faster than any woman before in history, and her teammate, Qu Yunxia, set a new women's world record in the 1,500 meters. In the preparations for the 2008 Summer Olympics in Beijing, the price of *Ophiocordyceps sinensis* skyrocketed. China, the host nation, won a record 100 medals and raked in more gold medals (51) than any other country. How much *Ophiocordyceps sinensis* contributed to that effort is a matter of conjecture.

What's not up for debate is how *Ophiocordyceps sinensis* has been described in Chinese and Tibetan traditional health volumes for many centuries, being recommended for the support of energy levels and endurance and a healthy immune system as well as the lungs and kidneys, according to research conducted by the *Journal of Ayurveda and Integrative Medicine.*

Today, *Ophiocordyceps sinensis* is being used to bio-transform herbs and foods to create the next generation of nutritional supplements.

3. Trametes versicolor

Trametes versicolor is the botanical name for the turkey tail mushroom, named for its colorful body. *Trametes versicolor* is world renowned for its ability to boost the immune system, according to a multiyear study funded by the National Institutes of Health (NIH).

Trametes versicolor is being tested at top institutions all over the world for its ability to support immune system health and vitality. In centuries past, *Trametes versicolor* has been used in Asia and Europe as a health-promoting tea.

4. Ganoderma lucidum

Here's another Asian fungus that has a long history of promoting health and longevity in China, Japan, and other Asian countries. In China, *Ganoderma lucidum* is the name for the lingzhi or reishi mushroom, and its health benefits are based largely on its traditional use and cultural mores, which is likely why it's been hailed as the "mushroom of immortality" or "supernatural mushroom."

Lingzhi has been the subject of Chinese life and art for thousands of years and is prized in Asia for its amazing health benefits. *Ganoderma lucidum* is known as a five-star Chinese adaptogen, signifying its supreme ability to ward off the damaging effects of stress and promote health and vitality.

Scientific studies have shown the efficacy of *Ganoderma lucidum* and its ability to support a healthy heart, upper respiratory system, and joint health and comfort while also supporting the immune system. But the latest research made headlines in 2015: scientists at the Chang Gung University in Taiwan believe that an extract of *Ganoderma lucidum* or reishi mushroom could help people lose weight, reduce inflammation, and lower the risk of type 2 diabetes by altering the bacteria in the gut.

"Our observations that [the mushroom extract] produces significant changes in the gut microbiota [microbiome] and the anti-obesity effects [of the extract] are transferable through fecal transplantation support the concept that obesity is associated with an altered gut microbiota," said the Chinese researchers.

5. *Hericium erinaceus*

This Latin phrase for "hedgehog" is also known as Lion's mane mushroom, which looks like a white pom-pom. These globular-shape mushrooms look nothing like the classic cap-and-stem button varieties you buy in the produce department.

Lion's mane mushrooms are being found in more and more gourmet grocery stores in this country as word slowly gets out about the nerve-supportive properties. A Huffington Post health story said, "Lion's mane mushrooms are increasingly studied for their neuro-protective effects. Two novel classes of Nerve Growth Factors (NGFs)—molecules stimulating the differentiation and re-myelination of neurons—have been discovered in this mushroom so far."

As promising research of this mushroom unfolds, lion's mane, or *Hericium erinaceus*, looks to be one of the more interesting nutritional superstars out there. They can be eaten when cooked in olive oil or coconut oil, but their chewy texture and taste is slightly reminiscent of seafood. *Hericium erinaceus* is being used more and more in nutritional supplements for its ability to support brain health.

6. *Bacillus subtilis*

I have a personal connection to this powerful microorganism that's pronounced *bah-sill-us subtle-is*, and that's because I first learned about this powerful microorganism from Peter Rothschild, an M.D. and Ph.D., who was a leading expert on human immune response and its relation to beneficial microorganisms. Dr. Rothschild was also one of the most interesting, enigmatic, and eccentric people I've ever met. He spoke seven languages and married as many times before his death about ten years ago. He definitely was a pioneer and a genius in the laboratory and in practice.

Dr. Rothschild made *Bacillus subtilis* the focus of much of his life's research and was one of the first to point out that beneficial microorganisms such as *Bacillus subtilis* dramatically benefit the human body's immune system even though they don't normally take up residence in the human gastrointestinal tract or are found in common foods consumed by Americans. The rod-shaped *Bacillus subtilis* bacteria is naturally found in soil and on vegetation.

I first heard of *Bacillus subtilis* when I was in San Diego during my health journey in the mid-1990s. My father had done some research and believed that *Bacillus subtilis* could help in my quest to improve my digestive and immune system health. Dad also had me read several articles and studies from Dr. Rothschild supporting his contention that *Bacillus subtilis* could do wonders for the gut and immune system. I would have to take it in supplement form because it wasn't found in common edible foods, although I would later learn that the fermented Asian soy food natto and the Nigerian fermented foods ogiri and dadawa are excellent sources of this powerful microbe.

Americans are generally not familiar with natto, which is made from fermented boiled soybeans and has a pungent aroma and taste that can be a stumbling block in this country. I recommend adding a dollop of natto over rice because research has found that both vitamin K_2 and a powerful enzyme named nattokinase are found within this extraordinary condiment. Vitamin K_2 and nattokinase contain cardiovascular protective qualities because they decrease the body's abilities to form blood clots. A growing body of science links vitamin K_2 (found in natto) and vitamin K_1 (found in leafy green vegetables) to benefiting bone and brain health.

Beans, legumes, and seeds fermented with *Bacillus subtilis* are the only foods where you find vitamin K_2 in its MK-7 form, nattokinase. When natto is consumed, for example, the *Bacillus subtilis* microorganisms travel down into the stomach, where potent gastric acids are waiting to burn up these beneficial microorganisms. *Bacillus subtilis,* however, is impervious to stomach acids.

After successfully marching through the stomach, *Bacillus subtilis* moves into the small and large intestines, where they attach themselves to the intestinal walls. *Bacillus subtilis* multiplies like crazy, and within a short period of time, the beneficial microorganisms populate—or colonize—the entire length of the gastrointestinal tract.

Bacillus subtilis also performs these tasks inside the gastrointestinal tract:

- promotes regular bowel function and helps maintain an already healthy immune system, both of which are beneficial to overall health

- maximizes the benefits of a healthy diet by supporting normal absorption and assimilation of nutrients in the gut

- helps support the normal gastrointestinal balance of good and potentially harmful bacteria and promotes regular bowel function

- supports the normal immune reaction of intestinal cells

- crowds out bacterial pathogens and maintains healthy gut flora

- communicates with intestinal cells to maintain gut barrier function

While my diet of raw goat's milk, raw sauerkraut, organic fruits and vegetables, and wild-caught fish helped me immensely in San Diego, I believe that taking *Bacillus subtilis* in a supplement form was the final piece of the health puzzle for me.

THE ULTIMATE TRANSFORMATION SYSTEMS

In this chapter, I've introduced four fungi and two bacteria as "agents of transformation" for our bodies. Over the last two years, my team and I have discovered two processes to radically transform foods and herbs using the ancient wisdom of fermentation with a modern twist. The Microbiome Transformation System utilizes beneficial bacteria such as *Bacillus subtilis* and *Lactobacillus plantarum* in a five-step potentiation process that includes:

1. Nutrient infusion

2. Active germination

3. Thermal liberation

4. Live fermentation

5. Frequency photon harmonization

These five steps result in *real* food NewTrients that are not mixed but instead are fused together by nature to become one living biomass.

I've always been a fan of fermentation and have formulated functional foods and nutritional supplements containing these types of ingredients in the past, but never at this level of complexity, which results in such a complete and effective fusion by nature. These processes have come from an evolution of my understanding of how to take the best foods on the planet and get the most out of them.

The process takes time, and it takes the right shepherding—kind of like being a coach and finding a great athlete and molding that person into an Olympic gold medal winner. That's really what we're trying to do—take something with great promise and unlock its full potential. I hope that our research and development in the area of fermentation will result in powerful foods, beverages, and nutritional supplements that can one day become a part of your daily diet and lifestyle.

Until that time, I encourage you to make fermented foods and beverages a significant part of your daily diet by experimenting with some homemade fermentation. Or, if you're not ready for that culinary adventure right away, consider purchasing live, organic fermented foods and/or nutritionals from your local health food store.

For more information on fermented foods and beverages and supplements, including DIY recipes and some of my favorite brands, visit www.PlanetHealThyself.com.

4

Eat Organic

My parents, Herb and Phyllis Rubin, were part of the counter-culture hippie generation that came of age in the late Sixties. They were teenagers and dating each other when they heard about a big concert being held on Max Yasgur's farm in upstate New York. They made the trek to Woodstock and joined 500,000 flower children for three days of peace and music that defined an era.

When my father enrolled at New York University—remember, he grew up in Long Island with Papa Jerry and Grandma Ann—he was a pre-med student who knew where he was going in life: medicine. My father, an excellent student who skipped two grades and started college at sixteen, was in the midst of applying to several medical schools when he happened to thumb through a magazine called *Prevention*, a healthy lifestyle periodical. His eyes spotted an advertisement from a school looking to train a "new breed" of doctors. He was on the med school track and a bit of a nonconformist, so when my intrigued father learned that the National College of Naturopathic Medicine was looking for students interested in treating patients from a whole different perspective than so-called "conventional medicine," something about pursuing a natural approach to medicine appealed to Dad's sensibilities.

When he delved further into naturopathy, Dad learned that the roots of naturopathic medicine could be traced back to the teachings of Hippocrates, Galen, and Paracelsus but had died out in the United States in 1954 with the closure of the last naturopathic medical school. The founding of the National College of Naturopathic Medicine two years later in Wichita, Kansas, however, resurrected naturopathic medical education, and the school was looking for interested students just like him.

That single advertisement in *Prevention* magazine changed the direction of my father's career path, as well as his life, when he decided to apply to the National College of Naturopathic Medicine. (The name has since been changed to the National College of Natural Medicine.) After receiving acceptance, he and Mom moved to Kansas in the mid-1970s for his first year of school. A little more than a year later, the school moved just outside of Portland, Oregon, and my parents relocated as well.

In the summer of 1975, Dad was taking a course in obstetrics and gynecology while Mom was in her final weeks of pregnancy with me. The way my father saw things, this was a chance for some hands-on experience.

When Mom's time came due and the contractions intensified, Dad and three other naturopathic students came over to the house to help perform the delivery. You could say that I was born with a silver sprout in my mouth because my back-to-nature, health-nut parents built their diet around farm-to-fork fruits and veggies purchased at a local co-op they co-founded. Sometime during my infancy, I could no longer tolerate Mom's breast milk, so they fed me goat's milk mixed with carrot juice in my bottle.

My parents didn't consume any dairy or meat products, however, because they were following a vegan lifestyle. This was back in the days before the term *vegan* came into vogue. Actually, they did consume some honey, so maybe they were "beegans." At any rate, that's the way I was raised for the first four years of my life until the day Grandma Rose sneaked me a chicken leg.

That opened the floodgates. You see, Mom had become pregnant with my younger sister, Jenna, and began to crave animal foods. When she and I started consuming animal foods during her pregnancy, my father soon followed suit.

Growing up, we moved several times before settling in South Florida's Palm Beach Gardens where I started second grade. I quickly learned that I was the odd kid in the neighborhood because I didn't eat the junk food my classmates wolfed down—potato chips, store-bought cookies, and ice cream bars. Whenever my school pals asked why I didn't have a piece of birthday cake at a classroom celebration, I'd shrug my shoulders and say, "I eat only organic foods."

In the mid-1980s, organic foods were just starting to come into their own as more and more parents and individuals became aware of the danger of eating fruits and vegetables coming from fields sprayed with pesticides. Their concern about the safety and nutritional value of conventionally grown foods motivated them to look for produce labeled as "organic." The term *organic* was coined in the 1950s by J.I. Rodale, the founder and publisher of *Prevention* magazine, who pioneered the idea that food grown without harmful chemicals was better for people and the planet.

By and large, organic farmers had their hearts in the right places, but there were a few growers eager to jump on the organic bandwagon and willing to cut corners on the production, handling, processing, and packaging of their "organic" agricultural products. There were no federal standards for what constituted organic food at the time or certification of farms. Instead, a patchwork of state laws lent a "Wild, Wild, West" atmosphere to the organic food industry.

Congress, feeling heat from its constituents to set national standards, passed the Organic Foods Protection Act in 1990. The legislation said that for any food to be called organic, it had to be grown without chemical fertilizers and pesticides. Animals had to be raised without antibiotics and growth hormones and given some access to the outdoors.

Turned out there were some exceptions—there always are because the devil is in the details. New legislation was needed, but it wasn't until 2001 that Congress passed a law giving the U.S. Department of Agriculture the power to establish federal standards that producers and handlers must follow in order to be certified organic and what organic food manufacturers are allowed to put on their packaging.

For shoppers, a green-and-white **USDA Organic** seal on single-ingredient foods like meat, eggs, and cheese means that the foods are 100 percent organic. For multi-ingredient foods such as beverages, snacks, and other processed foods, a classification system indicates the following:

- **100% Organic** means that foods bearing this label are made with 100 percent organic ingredients.

- **Organic** means this product contains 95 percent to 99 percent organic ingredients.

- **Made with Organic Ingredients** means at least 70 percent of the ingredients are organic and the remaining

30 percent do not include any biotechnological crops that had been genetically modified, meaning that scientists fiddled with the plant's genetic composition to boost crop yields or resistance to certain pests.

The USDA also set standards that growers have to follow to be certified organic. For fruits or vegetables, organic means the crop is grown without the use of most synthetic and petroleum-derived pesticides and fertilizers, antibiotics, genetic engineering, irradiation, and sewer sludge for three consecutive years. The reason I used the descriptor *most* is because the USDA's **Organic** label on multi-ingredient foods doesn't necessarily mean zero pesticides or herbicides; the non-organic 5 percent could be sprayed with pesticides and herbicides. There are about 200 non-organic substances producers can add to the fields or the food without losing the organic claim.

On the meat and dairy side, organic meats have to come from animals that eat 100 percent organic feed without any animal by-products; for dairy cows, the whole herd has to have eaten organic feed for the previous twelve months. There are loopholes that you can drive a cattle transport truck through, however.

Here's a case in point. In 2010, the USDA announced a new rule on access to pasture for organic ruminant animals (cows, sheep, and goats). Called an "enhancement" to the National Organic Standards, the new rules laid out these additional requirements:

- Animals must graze in pasture during the grazing season, which must be at least 120 days per year.

- Animals must obtain a minimum of 30 percent dry matter intake from grazing pasture during the grazing season.

- Livestock are exempt from the 30 percent dry matter intake requirement during the finish feed period, not to exceed 120 days. Livestock must have access to pasture during the finishing phase—or fattening up—prior to going to the slaughterhouse. During this period, the cattle can be fed just about anything, including grains or corn-based feed—as long as it's organic.

What this means is that the cattle aren't fattened up for the last few months of their lives from eating grasses in the field, but their steaks and hamburger meat can still be labeled "organic."

That's why, as I like to remind people, when it comes to organic livestock raised for meat, it's not so much how they start, it's how they finish.

LET'S TURN BACK THE CLOCK

So that's where we are, in a nutshell, with federal definitions of organic food. If it was up to me, I prefer a simpler definition that cuts to the heart of what organic food is all about:

Organic is the original way to grow and raise food.

Up until World War II, crops and animals were raised pretty much as they had been since biblical times—organically and sustainably, meaning a system of farming in which the animals ate a pasture-based diet and the farmlands maintained and replenished soil fertility without the use of toxic pesticides and NPK fertilizers. On the fishing side, fish were not pulled from the ocean faster than they could reproduce or caught in ways that destroy other sea life or undersea habitat.

Sure, mechanized machinery made agriculture much more efficient, and fishing techniques became more sophisticated, but when our grandparents were born—which isn't that long ago—our foods were grown organically and sustainably in a way that benefited the environment. There was no need to have an "Earth Day" every April 22. Every day was "Earth Day."

That all changed as chemistry made impressive strides during the Industrial Age from the late 1800s to the early 1900s, a fast-changing time when scientists discovered biochemical reactions regarding the properties, composition of, and changes in matter. New instruments and techniques made it possible to determine the molecular structure of elements in nature, and the changes that occurred between substances were shown graphically by chemical reactions.

For instance, a chemical compound called dichlorodiphenyltrichloroethane was first synthesized in 1874 by German scientist Othmar Zeidler, but no real use was found until 1939 when a Swiss chemist named Paul Müller discovered that dichlorodiphenyltrichloroethane—better known by its acronym DDT—made for a useful insecticide. Müller coated the inside of a glass box with this white, odorless powder and filled it with houseflies. Nothing happened at first, but when Müller returned the next morning, the flies were deader than doornails.

More tests were conducted by Müller, who worked for Geigy, a pharmaceutical and chemical company in Basel. DDT turned out to be a very effective insecticide. When World War II broke out, Switzerland declared its neutrality, and Geigy sold tons of DDT to the Germans and the Allies. Nazi Germany used DDT to boost food production, and Allies found that DDT protected troops and civilians from insect-borne diseases like malaria and typhus.

There's no doubt that DDT saved millions of lives and helped eradicate malaria in many countries. In India, at war's end in 1945, malaria infected an estimated 75 million and killed 800,000. In a few short years, that dropped dramatically to just a fraction of those numbers—a mere few thousand deaths.

In the post-war era, DDT became the gold standard for insecticides. A full-page advertisement in *Time* magazine in 1947 showed a group of cartoon animals, vegetables, and people singing in three-part harmony, "DDT is good for me-e-e!" The ad copy read, "The great expectations held for DDT have been realized. During 1946, exhaustive scientific tests have shown that, when properly used, DDT kills a host of destructive insect pests, and is a benefactor of all humanity."

DDT was hailed everywhere as a miracle pesticide. In 1948, Paul Müller was awarded the Nobel Prize for Physiology and Medicine for the way the insecticidal qualities of DDT saved millions from death to malaria, typhus, and yellow fever. People patted themselves on the back because modern science was responsible for taming some of the most devastating and infectious killers on the planet.

The ink on Müller's Nobel Prize certificate was barely dry, however, when scientists began noticing that the common housefly was developing an immunity to the pesticide. When the World Health Organization started a program in 1955 to eradicate malaria worldwide, increasing resistance from mosquitoes carrying the malaria parasite became a problem. What happened is that the few insects that survived bred, and their offspring proved more resistant to the effects of DDT. This necessitated various new pesticides, to which the insects eventually became resistant. Scientists also began finding high levels of DDT in fish, seals, whales, and crustaceans.

But it wasn't until the release of Rachel Carson's groundbreaking book, *Silent Spring*, published in 1962, that the tide of public opinion turned against DDT. Carson outlined the environmental disasters left in its wake, most notably the pesticide's impact on birds of prey. The author argued that DDT made bird eggshells thinner, leading to egg breakage and embryo death and severely harming bird reproduction. She also implied that DDT caused cancer in humans.

Environmentalists picked up the banner and fought to have DDT banned. After years of lobbying, they were successful in 1972 when the United States outlawed the use of DDT, and many countries adopted the same prohibition as well.

IN WIDE USE TODAY

Even though DDT was like the canary in a coal mine—a warning about the risks to the environment and our health from the use of pesticides—that didn't slow down the use of pesticides and herbicides in modern agriculture.

Today, dozens and dozens of various pesticides and herbicides are widely used. They are viewed as the only effective means of controlling disease-causing organisms, weeds, or insect pests, and Big Agriculture says that without important crop protection and pest control, U.S. food production would decline, many fruits and vegetables would be in short supply, and the price of food would rise.

Those may be valid talking points, but there's no way around the fact that pesticides are hazardous to one's health and horrible for the environment. The U.S. Environmental Protection Agency (EPA) had this to say:

> The [negative] health effects of pesticides depend on the type of pesticide. Some, such as the organophosphates and carbamates, affect the nervous system. Others may irritate the skin or eyes. Some pesticides may be carcinogens [cancer-producing]. Others may affect the hormones or endocrine system.

You don't have to read between the lines to understand that pesticides are harmful to humans. They *kill* what they are designed to kill because of their toxic nature, but the pests that survive reproduce, which starts the cycle all over again, and new, more powerful and, in turn, dangerous pesticides have to be created. Keep in mind that weeds also develop more resistant varieties. It's the law of unintended consequences in full swing.

We know the most commonly applied pesticides are:

- neonicotinoids, which kill insects

- herbicides, which kill weeds (think Roundup)

- rodenticides, which kill field mice and rodents

- fungicides, which kill fungi, mold, and mildew

Neonicotinoid pesticides are being studied for their role in the huge rise in honeybee losses that started in 2006. Bees have been dying off in record numbers in recent years, and managed honeybee colonies have recently suffered an annual loss of 42 percent, according to the U.S. Department of Agriculture. The majority of soybean, corn, canola, and sunflower seeds planted in the U.S. are sprayed with neonicotinoid pesticides, which travel through the plants and kill insects looking for a free lunch—but they also take out innocent pollinators such as bees and butterflies. A Harvard study released in 2014 reported that there is "convincing evidence" that neonicotinoid pesticides used on crops are linked to colony collapse disorder (CCD), a phenomenon in which adult bees simply disappear from their hives.

If dealing with pesticides wasn't enough, honeybees have also been hit by parasites and viruses sweeping through their colonies. A lack of diversity in single-crop monoculture is seen as another factor for the startling loss of millions of honeybees in the U.S. in recent years. The die-off of bees has *catastrophe* written all over it because bees pollinate 70 of the 100 different crops that make up 90 percent of the world's diet. Without bees doing their job, we won't have apples, onions, avocados, carrots, mangos, lemons, limes, cantaloupe, zucchini, eggplant, cucumbers, celery, kale, broccoli, and summer squash.

Yet the losses to the honeybee population continue to mount. Beekeepers who bring hives into fields from Pennsylvania to California may not have enough bees to pollinate trees and crop, leaving us a world with much less food. The tremendous losses of bees should be creating a buzz.

And still, the beat goes on in our pesticide-sprayed fields. According to the EPA, U.S. farmers used 516 million pounds of pesticides in 2008 (the latest year for data). Corn, soybeans, cotton, wheat, and potatoes account for 80 percent of pesticide use, but King Corn ranks number one and received 39 percent of pesticides used in 2008.

And guess what conventionally grown cattle eat for most of their lives: grain-based feeds made from corn and soy.

Actually, make that corn and soy treated with pesticides.

Raising livestock on various pesticide-treated grains is the equivalent of raising children on rotten candy because their stomachs are designed to receive pasture (grasses, legumes, forbs, and herbs) that is chewed and put through a wash-and-rinse cycle before being thoroughly digested.

Cattle are rarely pasture-fed and finished these days, however, unless they are raised for the organic and/or grass-fed marketplace. Instead, ranchers and cattlemen feed their conventionally raised livestock a formulated ration of grains mixed with corn, soy, and silage with a mishmash of antibiotics and hormones (although these synthetic additives are sometimes injected) to put on massive amounts of weight and prevent the cattle from getting sick or help them recover from an illness.

This use of antibiotics and hormones is routine and widespread in the meat-producing industry. According to the Grace Factory Farm Project, an estimated 80 percent of *all* antibiotics produced in the United States are fed to cattle, poultry, and pigs to compensate for the unsanitary and deplorable living conditions on "factory farms" that confine thousands of animals in impossibly cramped conditions, some with zero access to sunlight, fresh air, or natural movement.

Cattle usually have more space to roam around massive feed-lots, but not much. When cattle are transported to a new stock-yard, they are usually stressed by the experience and have weakened immune systems, meaning they are high risk. If 10 percent of the herd becomes sick within a week, the entire group receives antibiotics as a precautionary measure.

Hormones for livestock are more cut and dry—nearly all beef cattle entering feedlots and dairy operations are given hormone implants *and* anabolic steroids to promote faster growth before they're turned into rib-eyes and flank steak. Every pound that a head of cattle gains fattens the bottom line, as does every extra pint of coming from the udders of dairy cows. Even though the U.S. Food and Drug Administration has set "acceptable daily intakes" (ADIs) for these animal drugs, it's up to the producers to follow them.

The antibiotics fed to animals are similar to the antibiotics given to humans, which means the evolution of antibiotic-resistance bacterial strains is a serious public health threat. Growth hormones used to boost milk production and finishing weight become part of our food and have been studied for their links to all sorts of maladies, from increased risk for breast cancer and prostate cancer to the onset of early puberty in girls. While the scientific community is not ready to declare definite links, there's plenty of smoke clouding the issue.

One area where the research is more solid is the link between chemical toxins and fish. Researchers have found concentrations of polychlorinated biphenyls, a group of chemical compounds used in making paint, ink, dye, and hydraulic fluids, in the fatty tissues of fish around the globe. Metallic particles of mercury are especially prevalent in canned tuna.

Here's where I come down: each time you sit down for a steak dinner or pan-fried fish, remember that *you are what they ate.* If you've been consuming conventionally grown produce and meats all your life, then you've likely accumulated various toxins and chemicals and built up a "body burden." Pesticide residues are stored in your fatty tissues, where it can take months or years for these toxins to be eliminated from our system—and they can do plenty of damage in the meantime.

Last year, while driving to a meeting of progressive organic food and nutrition companies held in Oakland, California, I was on a highway near Fresno when I encountered what may have been the worst stench that had ever passed by my nostrils. This stink lasted for nearly twenty minutes as I noticed a massive conventional cattle-raising operation that housed what looked like tens of thousands of cows. What I didn't see was a single patch of pasture or even a blade of grass.

The issue of how we produce animal food greatly affects the health of our planet. More than 70 percent of U.S. cattle are raised in industrial feedlots, where they are fattened up before a one-way trip to the slaughterhouse. Packed in tightly and standing on a mixture of bare dirt and muck, the cattle don't have much room to move around. They produce tons of waste, which is dumped into huge "manure lagoons" that pass potentially toxic substances into our soil and groundwater.

As the effluent decomposes, these mountains of manure emit harmful gases and pollute the surrounding soil and water systems. Major storms result in overflows. When the waste is fully decomposed, it's often shipped to neighboring farms as fertilizer that certainly does *not* heal the planet.

It behooves us to be responsible for the way we treat the land by not polluting it and by managing it well for future years. Contrast the way conventional cattle are raised and their diet of grain-based feeds, usually made with a base of soy or corn, and pasture-raised cattle that graze on grasslands and even marginal land that doesn't have any other agricultural worth.

Jared Stone, author of *Year of the Cow: How 240 Pounds of Beef Built a Better Life for One American Family*, pointed out recent research that suggests that properly managed grass-fed cattle can help capture and store carbon in grassland soil. "In addition to making the soil more nutrient rich and better able to hold water, one study found this process happening at a rate that could actually help offset the rise in atmospheric carbon dioxide. It also showed that properly managed cattle pastures had levels of soil organic matter comparable with those of native forests."

Alan Savory, a biologist and former member of the Rhodesian Parliament, gave a "TED talk" at a recent Technology, Entertainment, and Design conference, asking the audience, "What are we going to do? There is only one option, I'll repeat to you, only one option left to climatologists and scientists, and that is to do the unthinkable, and to use livestock, bunched and moving, as a proxy for former herds and predators, and mimic nature. There is no other alternative left to mankind."

Stone and Savory raise some good points. As someone who raises cattle myself, I know that grass-fed cattle are better for healing the planet than raising cattle conventionally. Our cattle actually become a healthy part of the larger ecosystem.

ORGANIC FARMING IS TOPS

Organic farming is better for the planet, too, as you would expect. A thirty-year study by the Rodale Institute—the same folks behind *Prevention* magazine—came to the following conclusions:

- Yields from organic farming match yields from conventional farming.

- Organic farming outperforms conventional farming in years of drought.

- Organic farming systems build rather than deplete soil organic matter, making it a more sustainable system.

- Organic farming uses 45 percent less energy and is more efficient.

- Conventional farming produces 40 percent more greenhouse gases.

- Organic farming systems are more profitable than conventional.

The positives of eating organically raised foods that benefit our health and the health of the planet are enormous and life-changing. A comprehensive analysis and peer-reviewed study published in the *British Journal of Nutrition* confirmed what would appear to be a slam dunk: organic fruits and vegetables are not just less toxic but they are actually more nutritious than conventional produce.

The difference between organic and conventional produce was so striking, the researchers said, that switching to an all-organic diet might be the nutritional equivalent of adding one or two daily servings of fruits and vegetables to your diet. "The crucially important point about this research is that it shatters the myth that how we farm does not affect the quality of the food we eat," said Helen Browning, chief executive of the Soil Association.

In another study published in *The Journal of Applied Nutrition*, researchers purchased both organically and conventionally grown apples, potatoes, pears, wheat, and sweet corn in the western suburbs of Chicago over a two-year period and analyzed these foods for their mineral contents. Four to fifteen samples were taken for each food group.

On a per-weight basis, average levels of essential minerals were much higher in organically grown versus conventionally grown food. The organically grown food averaged 63 percent higher in calcium, 78 percent higher in chromium, 118 percent higher in magnesium, 178 percent higher in molybdenum, 91 percent higher in phosphorus, 125 percent higher in potassium, and 60 percent higher in zinc. And one more item to consider: organically raised food averaged 29 percent lower in mercury—a toxic metal—than the conventionally raised food.

Organic fruits and vegetables are bursting with flavor, have more "pop," and are flat-out better tasting than conventional food. Organic meat such as grass-fed beef and free-range chicken can have a definite earthy, grassy flavor but are generally leaner, more nutritious meats. Still, grass-fed beef can be wonderfully juicy and tender.

I can't really speak to the taste differences between grass-fed meat and conventionally produced meat because I can count the times I've knowingly eaten non-organic beef on two hands. Then I noticed that the Huffington Post conducted a blind taste test comparing a burger made with grain-fed supermarket beef versus one made with grass-fed beef, both 85 percent lean. Here's what reporter Julie R. Thomson wrote about the results:

Before we began the taste test, we worried that people wouldn't be able to taste the difference between regular and grass-fed beef. "How different could they be?" we wondered. We were *so* wrong. Every single editor was able to taste which burger was made with grass-fed beef, and they were almost 100 percent unanimous as to which one made the better burger. We learned firsthand that the price tag is worth it, people. Grass-fed beef makes for a significantly better tasting burger.

If you're still eating conventionally grown beef, I invite you to do a taste test—or just go out and buy yourself a couple of pounds of grass-fed beef. Yes, organic, grass-fed meat is more expensive, but the health benefits *and* the taste will make your investment pay off from the very first bite.

THE JOYS OF ORGANIC FOOD

I realize I'm a blessed person in many ways: my parents raised me right when it came to feeding me a diet that included organic foods.

What a gift I received—the joy of eating earth's bounty in the form of organic fruits, vegetables, dairy, meats, and wild-caught fish. Now that I'm a father, I can't explain how much it means to me to see my six children growing up healthy and *wanting* to eat nutritious, organically grown foods. I really believe that if you offered my kids junk food, they would politely say, "No, thank you," or at least inquire whether the food was organic.

I'm raising my children on a diet of healthful foods grown organically, foods that God created for us to eat in a form that's healthy for the body. I've eaten this way all my life and have walked the talk. A hidden camera crew from TMZ would get bored rather quickly trying to "catch" me sneaking a candy bar or grabbing a handful of potato chips at a Super Bowl party.

I *prefer* the taste of organic foods and the way they fill me with vitality. I love the flavors of organic fruits, vegetables, dairy, and meats, and you will, too.

When I go a health food store or a farmers market, I shop for:

- a wide array of organically grown fruits and vegetables

- healthy dairy products such as grass-fed butter

- healthy red meats including organic grass-fed beef, lamb, venison, and bison

- cold-water fish caught in the wild, such as sockeye salmon

- pasture-raised chicken and eggs

- whole grains such as amaranth, millet, buckwheat, and quinoa

- sprouted nuts and seeds

My wife, Nicki, and I enjoy building family dinners that begin with a healthy salad (romaine lettuce, radicchio, escarole, and endive) with tomatoes, celery, red onions, peppers, and avocados. Then one of us will bake, grill, or brown in a saucepan (with coconut oil) our protein: organic grass-fed meat, free-range chicken, or wild-caught fish. We adorn our plates with healthy vegetables such as spinach, broccoli, cauliflower, or sweet potatoes as well as a gluten-free, high-antioxidant grain such as black quinoa.

SALES ARE UP

The message that organic foods give your body a greater quantity of essential nutrients, are grown or raised without pesticides and synthetic chemicals, and are easy on the calories has seeped slowly but surely into the culture. What's happened over the last twenty-five years is nothing short of amazing: the market for organic foods has grown dramatically in ways that no one could have predicted. The most telling statistic is that U.S. sales of organic food and beverages grew from $1 billion in 1990 to $28.4 billion in 2012, a nifty 2,700 percent increase.

I'm heartened by the greater availability of organic produce, dairy, and meat products today. Natural food groceries such as Whole Foods, Sprouts, Natural Grocers, Earth Fare, New Seasons, and Fresh Thyme Farmers Markets are popping up in cities and suburbs around the country, and local independent health food stores are going strong. Even major grocery chains and warehouse clubs have dedicated entire aisles to organic foods.

While organic food sales have been showing double-digit increases from year to year, they still account for only about 4 percent of total food sales, and the market for grass-fed beef is less than 4 percent of all U.S. beef sales. That means the other 96 percent is still coming from shopping carts filled with conventionally grown fruits and vegetables, cellophane-wrapped packets of conventionally raised beef, chicken, and farm-raised fish, and assorted boxes and packages of processed foods such as breakfast cereals, bakery items, lunchmeats, frozen meals, and sweet treats.

The reason why many families are stuck in the conventional side of the aisle is because of their cost. I get that. The economy has been stagnant in recent years and household income has gone down. Many parents are working extra jobs to keep food on the table and the rent or mortgage paid.

Organic fruits, vegetables, meats, and dairy products are more expensive, generally anywhere from 20 percent to 100 percent more than conventionally grown and raised groceries. But there are ways to get a lot of organic bang for your buck:

- **Stock up at sale time.** Yes, even organic products go on sale at health food grocery stores.

- **Shop at farmers markets.** Food that's grown, produced, and sold locally is a great way to help the planet heal itself, and without middlemen between you and the grower, the prices can be excellent. Farmers market produce tastes better than fruits and vegetables that have traveled thousands of miles from farm to plate.

- **Eat organic food instead of going out to a restaurant.** Yes, this means time spent preparing and cooking organic foods, but eating organic food is cheaper than taking the family to a fast-food place or "fast casual" restaurant—and much healthier, of course. A family of four would have to pay a minimum of $20 to $25 for a meal out, but you could pay for a wonderful home-cooked meal complete with organic, grass-fed beef or wild-caught fish for that amount—even less. But if you're interested in eating out, search for local organic restaurants as more and more of them are opening their doors in major and even smaller cities all across the U.S.

- **Eating organic is cheaper than going on a special diet.** And there's a good chance you'll lose extra pounds that wouldn't come off with any other diet.

- **If you're taking nutritional supplements, shop organic as well.** Surveys suggest that 40 percent to 70 percent of Americans consume nutritional supplements, so look for products that are certified organic (check for the USDA seal) as more and more leading brands are taking the giant leap and producing nutritional formulations using organic ingredients.

When you get down to the nitty-gritty, the decision to eat organic foods boils down to what's important to you. What you spend your money on shows where your interests lie and where your heart is.

Do you want to live a healthier life and leave a smaller footprint on the planet? Do you see organic foods as a down payment for your future and your health?

Let me leave you with little saying that puts everything in perspective:

You can pay the farmer now, or you can pay the doctor later.

For more information on eating organic, including recipes and sources of my favorite organic foods, beverages, and supplements, visit www.PlanetHealThyself.com.

5

Say No to GMO

I WAS LIVING THE DREAM, DOING EXACTLY WHAT I HOPED I'D BE DOING ever since I recovered from severe health challenges during my college years.

But never in my wildest fantasies did I ever believe that twelve short years later I would find myself relaxing on dark blue leather couches inside a forty-five-foot Prevost tour bus while I crisscrossed the country, presenting seminars at local health food stores, schools, and universities, visiting organic farms, conducting interviews with the media, and filming episodes for my TV show, *Perfect Weight America*.

On board our tour bus—wrapped with a red, white, and blue Perfect Weight America logo—was a camera crew that followed me everywhere. It was like living in a reality show, being on the road promoting my new book, *Perfect Weight America*, and sharing my message of healthy eating, nutritional supplementation, and emotional health during a coast-to-coast adventure across the United States. Over six months, we would travel 40,000 miles and make stops in more than 200 towns and cities.

One particular memory stands out. We were rolling through the verdant farmlands of the Midwest on a late springtime afternoon. Blue sky above and a green carpet of maturing crops as far as the eye could see.

From my comfortable couch, my mind wandered. I thought about how millions of green leaves and shoots were capturing the power of the sun through a process called photosynthesis. As the cropland came into full view, what looked like beautiful farmland from afar took on a different appearance altogether. I found myself envisioning my children's stolen future as everywhere I looked across the fruited plain, I saw genetically modified, monocrop agriculture dominating the landscape.

I knew that American agriculture had become "agribusiness," which is a commonly used term that defines how farming has evolved in the last fifty years. Market forces had changed the way we grow, transport, promote, and sell food in the marketplace. The first segment—the mom-and-pop family farm—had given way to large-scale, industrialized, and corporate-owned farming enterprises.

I understood *why* farming had evolved in this direction. In order to stay in business, farming operations must produce the biggest yields possible for the lowest price. If that means planting precision rows of the same crop for economy of scale, sending out crop dusters to lay down a pesticide mist to protect their investment, using herbicides to kill stubborn weeds, buying huge machinery that can reap the harvest more efficiently, or picking fruits and vegetables before they ripen (and then gassing them on their way to market), then that's what they were going to do to improve the bottom line.

The realization that this is what farming had come to saddened me.

I came to another bittersweet awareness that day: many farmers with ten, twenty, one hundred, or a thousand acres couldn't feed their own family because they planted a single crop—wheat, corn, potatoes, or soybeans—instead of having a mixed polyculture or permaculture farm growing multiple species. What they harvested was trucked to a grain elevator, where it was sold into market or exported to a populous country like China or Russia. The money they received for toiling in the fields was used to buy the same groceries and foods that everyone else buys in the nation's supermarkets. In other words, these farmers couldn't even feed their own families because of the way farming is practiced today—nor could they eat organically because their farms don't produce organic crops.

Plain and simple, food had become a manufactured commodity. Farmers had become part of an interconnected system in which huge food conglomerates transported the fruit of their labor to a far-off packaging factory, food manufacturing plant, or industrial bakery where their crops were stripped of vital nutrients, pumped up with additives, and laced with preservatives in the production of mass-produced and mass-marketed foods.

I experienced an epiphany in the stillness of my heart while rolling down the interstate from Nebraska to Iowa with literally the voice of God speaking to me: *Jordan, you need to farm your own food, for your family and to provide for as many others as you can. This is something you must do…for yourself, for your loved ones, and for the planet as your contribution to future generations.*

I kept this experience in the back of my mind when I visited dozens of organic farms and talked to these hard-working agrarians about the pressing problems they faced. While these devoted farmers had all the right intentions, I couldn't help but notice that a lack of resources kept many running a shoestring operation.

Back in Florida, I talked about my revelation with Nicki. After a lively discussion, she was on board. We both understood that buying a farm would represent a major change in the trajectory of our lives. Nicki was game. She saw the big picture. After searching for land all across America, we found just the right place in southern Missouri's Ozark Mountains.

Instead of simply writing about and lecturing on the problems with the American food supply, instead of complaining about the growing preponderance of genetically modified foods and ingredients lining the shelves of our nation's grocery stores, and instead of sitting on the sidelines, I decided to get in the game—and become part of the solution.

A PRIMER ON GM FOODS

Maybe you're heard of genetically modified (GM) foods. Maybe you're aware of the battle that's raging within the outer fringes of our country's populace pushing for truth in labeling and calling for a nationwide revolt against genetic modification. Or, you may be blissfully unaware of the planned assault on our food supply waged by multinational agribusiness corporations. A nationwide survey released by researchers at Rutgers University found that a little more than half (53 percent) of respondents said they knew very little about genetically modified foods, and one in four (25 percent) said they had never heard of them.

Genetically modified foods means that they are made from crops produced from genetically modified seeds infused with genetically modified organisms (GMO), meaning these growing or living things have been artificially manipulated through genetic engineering. The idea behind genetically modifying crops is that the seeds to produce dietary staples such as corn, soybeans, and even cotton can be altered by combining plant, animal, bacteria, and viral genes in ways that do not occur in nature or through traditional crossbreeding methods, also known as hybridization, in order to "improve" the plant.

Scientists believe that taking genes from one organism and inserting them into another makes the plants grow higher, larger, denser, and more resistant to insect infestation. While this is a laudable goal, the problem is that scientists are adding certain genes to seeds that weren't originally part of the equation, which is unnatural and changes the DNA of the crop. "You just can't get an elephant to mate with a corn plant," said Margaret Mellon of the Union of Concerned Scientists. "Scientists are making combinations of genes that are not found in nature."

The reason why scientists began tinkering with the genetic makeup of crops is because Monsanto, an agriculture biotech company, developed a powerful weed killer called Roundup in the 1970s that contained glyphosate, an agricultural herbicide. An idea formed among Monsanto scientists: *What if we could develop crops that would have a specific immunity or resistance to Roundup so that farmers could use our herbicide to kill all the weeds in their fields but leave the cash crop alone?*

Soybeans were the first large-scale crop to undergo genetic modification. Years of experimentation and testing resulted in the first fields of GM soybeans being planted in 1996, followed by corn in 1998, and then it was off to the races. More crops were genetically modified—cotton, sugar beets, and canola—and "fine-tuned" to produce an insecticide in every plant cell during the growing season.

Conventional farmers discovered that they liked GM seeds with this feature because their pesticide and herbicides costs dropped substantially. According to a report in *Capital Press*, a leading pro-agriculture publication, "A meta-analysis, which reviewed 147 other studies, found that by growing GM crops, farmers reduced pesticide costs by 37 percent. At the same time, farmers' profits increased by 68 percent."

The use of seeds altered with GMOs skyrocketed during the '00s as conventional farming adopted GM technology en masse, which resulted in significant economic advantages to farmers. Scientists in the agricultural industry, along with academic researchers, touted the benefits of genetically modified food, saying that without GM crops, there would be no way to feed a growing world population bursting at the seams.

But what about government oversight? What did the Environmental Protection Agency have to say?

Lawyers representing agribusiness argued that genetically modified organisms were simply extensions of normal plant breeding that occurs in nature, much like how a horticulturist would graft tissues from a rose stem onto another similar plant. That argument carried the day, which is the reason why no laws have been passed in Congress regarding the regulations of GMOs to this day. But what no one saw coming was that the U.S. Patent Office would allow corporations like Monsanto to patent their genetically modified seeds to protect their "intellectual property."

Nonetheless, as genetically modified crops gained widespread acceptance, they were hailed in the popular culture for:

- reducing the need for pesticides and herbicides (even though the plants themselves contain the herbicide glyphosate)

- reducing greenhouse emissions because GM crops require less tillage or plowing, thus less use of fossil fuels

- giving scientists the ability to manipulate foods to increase desirable components such as nutrients

- increasing food production in starving Third World countries

Twenty years after the first fields of genetically modified soybeans were planted, much of the arable land in the United States—more than 90 percent—is now planted with seeds containing genetically modified organisms. I would call that a near-total victory. Around the world, approximately 50 percent of farmlands are using GM seeds, and that percentage is growing. The production of GM seeds is a huge industry bringing in revenues in the tens of billions of dollars annually. Four global multinational corporations pretty much control the GMO market worldwide:

- Monsanto

- DuPont

- Dow Chemical

- Sygenta

All the agribusinesses except for Sygenta, a Swiss firm, are based in the United States, which is the world's leader in GM agriculture. Here's a breakdown of the major GM crops growing in the United States, according to the Center for Food Safety and the Non-GMO Project:

- corn (approximately 93 percent of the U.S. crop)

- soybeans (approximately 94 percent of the U.S. crop)

- cotton (approximately 96 percent of the U.S. crop, and cottonseed oil is often used in food products)

- sugar beets (approximately 94 percent of the U.S. crop)

- canola (approximately 90 percent of the U.S. crop, and canola oil is often used in food products)

- papaya (most of the Hawaiian crop)

- zucchini and yellow summer squash (approximately 25,000 acres are in production)

The switch from conventional to GM crops has happened in the blink of an eye—just twenty years. But at what cost to humans and to our planet?

The jury is still out, although I count myself among consumer advocates, environmental activists, and numerous scientists warning of an unforeseen environmental disaster with severe health and socioeconomic consequences. I've spoken several times with Jeffrey Smith, author of *Genetic Roulette: The Documented Health Risks of Genetically Engineered Foods* and *Seeds of Deception: Exposing Industry and Government Lies about the Safety of the Genetically Engineered Foods You're Eating,* and I appreciate the research and information-gathering he's done to warn the American public that foods with genetically modified ingredients are toxic and can open the door to allergic reactions, infertility, and digestive disorders, to name a few. Another danger is that the bacteria in our gut could pick up antibiotic-resistant genes found in many GM foods—and start to destroy beneficial microorganisms inside our digestive tracts.

Jeffrey, who famously quipped one time that GMO should stand for "God Move Over," offered this overview about the dangers of genetically modified crops:

We all know the stories of tobacco, asbestos, and DDT. Originally declared safe, they caused widespread death and disease. Although their impact was vast, most of the population was spared. The same cannot be said for sweeping changes in the food supply. Everyone eats; everyone is affected. The most radical change occurred when genetically modified crops were introduced…made possible by a technology whereby genes from one species are spliced into the DNA of other species.

Herbicide-tolerant soy, corn, cotton, and canola plants are engineered with bacterial genes that allow them to survive otherwise deadly doses of herbicides. This gives farmers more flexibility in weeding and gives the GM seed company more profit. When farmers buy GM seeds, they sign a contract to buy only that seed producer's brand of herbicide….

[Regarding GM foods], the FDA declared that GM crops are "Generally Recognized as Safe" (GRAS) as long as their producers say they are. Thus, the FDA does not require any safety evaluations or labeling of GMOs. A company can even introduce a GM food to the market without telling the agency.

I've stated consistently in my previous books that I will not purchase, or knowingly eat, foods produced from genetically modified ingredients and will continue to warn everyone who will listen of their potential dangers until we have a solid body of research regarding the short-term and long-term effects of eating GMO foods—and it doesn't look like that's happening any time soon.

Notice that I used the qualifier *knowingly*. Our family doesn't eat conventional foods very often, but on the rare occasions we do, we have *no way* of knowing if that product contained genetically modified components because GM ingredients do not have to be disclosed on food labels or menus at restaurants. Legislative bills requiring mandatory labeling of genetically engineered foods have been introduced in Congress, but nothing has been passed at the time of this writing. Two states, Connecticut and Maine, passed GM labeling laws in 2013, and Vermont's new law goes into effect in 2016. Bills have been introduced in two dozen other states.

While these are positive developments, it's a head-scratcher why GMOs are getting a free pass. Dr. Martha Herbert, a pediatric neurologist, brain development researcher, and assistant professor of Neurology at the Harvard Medical School, made this comment:

> Today the vast majority of foods in supermarkets contain genetically modified substances whose effects on our health are unknown. As a medical doctor, I can assure you that no one in the medical profession would attempt to perform experiments on human subjects without their consent. Such conduct is illegal and unethical. Yet manufacturers of genetically altered foods are exposing us to one of the largest uncontrolled experiments in modern history.

I'm not buying the argument that GMOs are safe. Governments in many developed countries around the world share a similar worldview, which explains why there are significant restrictions or outright bans on the production of GM crops in more than sixty countries, including all of the countries in the European Union as well as Japan and Australia. The concerns are so genuine that EU countries refuse the importation of GM foods and seeds from the U.S., which contributes to our trade imbalance and keeps more GM foods inside *our* country.

The United States is the outlier in terms of GMO acceptance and the reason why an estimated 75 percent of the processed foods in this country (breads, breakfast cereals, baked goods, soda, beer, vegetable oils, and even nutritional supplements) contain a potpourri of genetically modified ingredients.

I think the percentage is higher than that. In fact, I wouldn't be surprised if in the near future *all* processed foods have GM ingredients. I don't see how you could assume otherwise. If corn or soy is part of the ingredients list—and we know that more than 90 percent of corn and soy comes from genetically modified crops—then that food likely has genetically modified ingredients. And don't forget that many additives, preservatives, and natural flavors are derived from genetically modified corn and soy, so for all intents and purposes, these genetically modified ingredients are invisible to the American public.

The Non-GMO Project, an independent organization, has stepped into the vacuum created by the lack of leadership from federal agencies responsible for food safety. Believing that consumers should have access to clearly labeled GM food and products, the Non-GMO Project began an independent verification process of the GM content in foods and products.

While the Non-GMO Project cannot state with absolute certainty that any food or product is GMO-free—due to the limitations of testing methodology—shoppers like myself can feel very confident that what we're buying and consuming was not made with genetically modified ingredients if the Non-GMO Project Verified seal is on the packaging. Companies looking to receive the Non-GMO Project Verified seal must follow the project's standards of best practices and product testing conducted at various stages of production, anywhere from the field to the packaging facility.

The only other way to assure yourself that you're not eating GM foods is to purchase foods with the USDA Organic label as GMOs are prohibited from certified organic products. Under USDA rules, farmers are not allowed to grow produce from GM seeds, their animals cannot eat GM feed, and organic food producers can't use GM ingredients.

As of the writing of this book, the USDA is in the process of creating its own non-GMO labeling standards, which will operate in a similar fashion to the organic labeling program. This is a good start, but until mandatory nationwide GM labeling in enacted, the consumer will never be in the know and empowered to make an informed choice.

Without the stamps of approval from the USDA Organic or Non-GMO Project labels, or at the very least a non-GMO or GMO-free designation made by the brand of product your purchasing, your GM goose is cooked. Sure, the cattle, pigs, goats, and poultry we use for food or to make dairy products are not genetically modified, but as their animal feed is usually comprised of corn and/or soybeans that contain GMOs, you can assume that meat and dairy foods found in grocery markets or neighborhood restaurants do have genetically modified ingredients.

That popular breakfast flake cereal?

Made from genetically modified corn.

That loaf of bread you bought at a local bakery?

Made with canola oil or soybean oil, each containing GMOs.

That New York strip steak sizzling on your barbecue?

That prime cut came from cattle fed an abundance of genetically modified corn and soy, which tops the list of the Top Seven most common GMO foods, according to the Cornucopia Institute:

1. **Corn** is everywhere and is the breakfast of champions (as well as lunch and dinner) for our livestock. Author Michael Pollan, whom I enjoy reading, said, "Corn is what feeds the steer that becomes your steak. Corn feeds the chicken and the pig. Corn feeds the catfish raised in a fish farm. Corn-fed chickens lay the eggs. Corn feeds the dairy cows that produce milk, cheese, and ice cream. Chicken nuggets are really corn wrapped up in more corn. If you wash down your

chicken nuggets with almost any soft drink, you are drinking corn with your corn." There's a corny joke there somewhere, but GMOs are not something to laugh about.

2. **Soy** and hydrolyzed soy protein is in nearly 75 percent of products on supermarket shelves and nearly 100 percent of fast food.

3. Ever wonder where the name **canola oil** came from? Answer: **Can**adian **o**il **l**ow **a**cid, and I kid you not. This oil produced from the rapeseed plant is found in many baked goods.

4. Cottonseed oil, which comes from **cotton**, is another cheap vegetable oil that's used in salad dressings, mayonnaise, sauces, and marinades. Cottonseed oil ranks third in volume behind soybean and corn oil.

5. **Milk** is pumped out of the udders of black-and-white Holstein cows that eat corn-based GM feed.

6. Genetically modified **sugar beets** are late omers to the party, having been introduced in 2009. They're making up for lost time when a sugar is needed to sweeten a baked good.

7. Last is **Aspartame**, an artificial sweetener made from genetically modified bacteria; it is the sweetening agent known as NutraSweet and Equal. Long questioned for its possible link to certain cancers, Aspartame's checkered past caught up to it in 2015 when Pepsi dropped Aspartame because sales of Diet Pepsi had

fallen by more than 5 percent. Diet Coke, which also contains aspartame, decreased by more than 6 percent, but aspartame remains a key ingredient.

There are more genetically modified foods being grown than you'd think because with no labeling requirements, few realize they are eating them. For instance, I'd be willing to wager that your local grocery carries zucchini, yellow squash, and papaya grown from GM seeds. Meanwhile, biotech scientists are tucked away in their laboratories, toiling away on the next generation of GM foods.

We may see some attention-grabbing additions in the near future. In 2015, the U.S. Food and Drug Administration approved two varieties of genetically engineered apples and six varieties of genetically engineered potatoes. The FDA concluded that "these foods are as safe and nutritious as their conventional counterparts." What greatly concerns me even more is that the FDA still isn't willing to require companies to label the produce as being genetically modified.

Gratefully, the FDA has yet to approve the application for the first genetically modified animal food to enter the U.S. food supply. I'm talking about "AquaAdvantage salmon," an the Orwellian trade name for a genetically modified Atlantic salmon made from a growth hormone-regulating gene from a Pacific Chinook salmon, a "promoter" gene from a ray-finned fish known as an ocean pout, and 40,000 genes from an Atlantic salmon. The idea is producing a fast-growing fish that can be taken to market in sixteen to eighteen months instead of the customary three years.

I can't see how any of this GMO nonsense can do anything but harm our bodies and the planet. While proponents of GM foods believe they are riding the wave of the future, I'm worried that we may be unleashing a form of "agricultural asbestos" on the unsuspecting

American public. That's why my family and I continue to shop for organic, non-GMO fruit, vegetables, grains, and meats.

Besides, just on taste alone, organic foods have genetically modified crops beat by a country mile.

A CLOSING THOUGHT

In 2014, I was asked to speak at a homeschooling conference in St. Louis, so this looked like a good opportunity to take the family to the "big city." The Heal the Planet Farm at Beyond Organic Ranch is in a remote, unpopulated area of southern Missouri not far from the Arkansas state line.

While in St. Louis, our family visited the St. Louis Zoo. I've been to several zoos around the country, but the St. Louis Zoo was exceptional. Even better, admission was free. Some of the attractions, such as the sea lion show and the children's zoo, required a fee, however.

We purchased tickets on the tram to visit each section of the zoo, and at one of the stops, the driver said, "Welcome to the Monsanto Insectarium, which is having a special exhibition on butterflies this month."

My son, Joshua, who was nine at the time, blurted, "Monsanto? They're evil, Dad."

A few people turned in our direction with "shocked" expressions on their faces, but when you teach your children the truth, they tend to see the world in black and white and very little gray.

It was time to step off the tram, so we moved on, but what I would have said to those who overheard Joshua was that Monsanto and farmers who raise GM crops are *not* evil—far from it. Those behind the development of GM seeds and those raising crops from those seeds are simply doing what they believe to be their job, although I must note that company execs are driven largely by profits and have ignored many warnings on the dangers of GMOs. I believe, however, they are very misguided.

Listen, after diving into farming myself, I have a great appreciation for how difficult it is to get something to grow out of the ground, harvest it, and get it to your table, much less the market. When I'm at the Heal the Planet Farm, there isn't a day that goes by when I don't shovel, plant, or harvest something. That's why I marvel at how people can walk into a health food store and say, "Wow, organic blueberries are $4.99 a pint," or "This loaf of organic bread is really expensive." From my vantage point, I can't believe how relatively affordable organic foods are, given the time, effort, and energy that was put into producing them.

So I want to go easy on conventional farmers who are growing genetically modified crops, realizing that they are simply trapped in the agricultural system of degeneration. I prefer that market forces determine the fate of GM foods, just as those same forces moved Pepsi to stop using a toxic artificial sweetener called Aspartame. If you and I and all our friends start buying organic foods and consume more organic produce and organically raised meat and dairy than we did last week, last month, and last year, we send a message each time we hand our credit cards to the checkout clerk. Less of a demand for conventional foods made with GM crops means more biodiversity in plants, insects, and animals. More biodiversity means greater health for our bodies and the planet.

Biodiversity is a term that describes the number of different species that live within a particular ecosystem. The preservation of biodiversity should be a major goal for everyone. While living in California recently, I learned how almond growers are greatly concerned that the steady shrinkage of honeybees—which pollinate their trees—could mean the loss of their almond crops, which account for more than *80 percent* of the world's supply.

For the last decade, beehives across the country have been disappearing at alarming rates because of a mysterious mass die-off of honeybees that pollinate $30 billion worth of crops in the U.S. Scientists are struggling to find a reason for the so-called Colony Collapse Disorder (CCD), which has wiped out an estimated 10 million beehives. Scientists at the University of Maryland and the U.S. Department of Agriculture believe they've found the culprit: a witch's brew of pesticides and fungicides contaminating pollen that bees collect to feed their hives.

Pesticides, herbicides, fungicides…the rise of genetically modified foods…and a startling decrease in biodiversity…they all directly impact the planet. The only way we can turn things around is to change our buying habits—and make our views known.

Maybe a tipping point happened in early 2015 when Chipotle, the fast-casual restaurant chain that serves burrito bowls, soft tacos, and salads, announced that it is eliminating GMO-containing ingredients in the foods it serves. The chain said that some of its meat and dairy will still come from animals fed GMO grains, but the company was working on a solution for that, too. Soft drinks with high fructose corn syrup—another GM corn derivative—will continue to be on the menu, however. (Until patrons start asking for water.)

We'll have to see how it all plays out and if other restaurant chains or big food companies start moving to take GM ingredients out of their products. But what I'd like to see first is mandatory labeling of products so that consumers know if any ingredients come from genetically modified sources.

This will only happen if and when we refuse to consume foods or supplements containing GMOs. The only way to ensure this is to shop for foods and supplements that are free of GM crops and their derivatives altogether, or those labeled organic or non-GMO.

For more information on GMOs, including ways to get involved in the fight against GMOs and truth-in-labeling campaigns as well as sources of non-GMO foods, beverages, and supplements, visit www.PlanetHealThyself.com.

6

Go Gluten-Free

WHILE I WAS WRITING *Planet Heal Thyself,* I TOOK A GENETIC TEST through the website 23andMe. All I had to do was spit in a vial, dispatch the tube of saliva into the mail, and the lab team at 23andMe—named after the twenty-three pairs of chromosomes in a normal human cell— provided me with personal insight into my ancestry, genealogy, and inherited traits.

I already knew that I am of Jewish descent; both my parents and grandparents came from Jewish families. According to 23andMe, the genetic testing revealed that I was of 98 percent Ashkenazi Jewish descent. Genesis 10:3 describes how Ashkenaz was the son of Gomer, whose grandfather was Noah. The Ashkenzai Jews are believed to have migrated from the Middle East in the first century A.D. and settled in southern and eastern Europe, where they grew in numbers during the Middle Ages and beyond.

While it was fascinating to peek into my ancestral history, I was able to dig deeper into my personal genomics through LiveWello, which took my 23andMe lab results and determined that I was homozygous for a gene that predisposes me to gluten sensitivity or even intolerance. *Homozygous* comes from the Greek root *homo*, which means "same," and *zygote* is a cell created when two gametes (a sperm and an egg, in humans) come together.

Just because a lab test said I was predisposed to gluten sensitivity doesn't mean that my body will be reactive to gluten, but after dealing with severe digestive issues and inflammation in the past, I decided to take the plunge and go completely off gluten.

Gluten is the name for a protein found in wheat, rye, barley, and triticale (a hybrid of wheat and rye). The wheat varieties go by names such as durum, kamut, emmer, spelt, farina, farro, and einkorn. Gluten helps foods maintain their shape, acting like a glue that holds food together. The gluten protein, however, is highly inflammatory for some people and opens the door to a host of digestive, neurological, and immunological issues.

I, myself, have not consumed a lot of "intact" gluten over the years. When I've eaten gluten, it's usually been in the form of sprouted and sourdough whole-grain breads, whereby the processes of sprouting and/ or fermentation (sourdough) predigests much of the gluten. The germinating process or sour leavening helps break down gluten's "stickiness," so this allowed me to eat the occasional sandwich made from sprouted bread or dig into a plate of angel hair spelt pasta topped with organic tomato sauce. I also consumed heirloom grains such as einkorn, the world's most ancient wheat and completely unhybridized. The hybridization of wheat and the grain-centric culture we live in today is one of the reasons gluten can be a major challenge to your health.

Knowing this, and after receiving the results of my genetic testing, something told me it was time to say *sayonara*, *auf Wiedersehn*, and goodbye to gluten in 2015, so that's what I've done.

I don't believe I'm gluten intolerant, nor do I have celiac disease, a digestive and autoimmune disorder in which the small intestine is hypersensitive to gluten, leading to difficulty in digesting food. I'm not even certain that I have a gluten sensitivity, meaning that gluten gives me troubles every now and then in the form of abdominal pain, bloating, and diarrhea. What I do believe is that I have a genetic disposition to difficulties metabolizing gluten because of the circumstances and environmental challenges that I've experienced that have led to past issues related to my gut. Because I want to be free of inflammation and perform at my best, I've decided to take the gluten question off the table and avoid this protein completely for the time being.

Kicking the gluten habit puts me in good company. Seems like there's a story every week about a world-class athlete or famous celebrity who's kicked gluten to the curb. One of the latest is Mark Teixeira, the home run-slugging first baseman for the New York Yankees. (His Portuguese surname is pronounced *Te-share-ah.*) I've always liked the Bronx Bombers, probably because my parents grew up in the New York area.

Yankee fans know that Teixeira had suffered through a pair of injury-ridden seasons with wrist, hamstring, and lower-back injuries. One more subpar year, and the thirty-four-year-old first basemen could be out of baseball. Determined to stay on the field, Teixeira sought out answers and learned that going on a gluten-free diet may reduce inflammation in his body.

Bothered by swelling and soreness that compromised his chances of being in the starting lineup as well as his ability to turn on a baseball, Teixeira committed to a gluten-free diet before the start of the 2015 season. The results were everything that Teixeira and Yankee fans were hoping for as the veteran slugger positioned himself among the top home run leaders during the 2015 season and earned a midseason All-Star selection.

Dozens of top athletes have turned to gluten-free diets in the last few years. In the NFL, Drew Brees, the New Orleans quarterback, was diagnosed with severe food allergies in his twenties, along with his wife, Brittany. "I had started to feel really lethargic and just felt like I wasn't operating at the highest level," Brees said. "That's when we both went in for testing. Brittany and I both came back with sensitivities to dairy—milk, cheese, and yogurt—as well as gluten, and I was also allergic to some nuts. As you can imagine, I was shocked because I was consuming most of these things every day. And just to think how long I've had these sensitivities and had continued to feed them. I felt it was time for a change."

Endurance athletes have been jumping aboard the gluten-free bandwagon, too. Members of the Garmin team competing in the Tour de France cycling race have been gluten-free since 2008. Riders devour at least 8,000 to 9,000 calories in a twenty-four-hour period in order to pedal 150 miles a day, more than three times what most of us need. To help ensure that these elite racers don't "bonk" during competition, Tour de France riders traditionally carbo-load on mountains of pasta the night before a race—grains being the main source of carbohydrates. Carbs break down into glucose, which is the fuel the body draws upon during intense exercise.

Jonathan Vaughters, Garmin's founder and CEO, was concerned that the gluten caused bloating, stiffness, and gastrointestinal distress and theorized that his team would recover better from grueling stages if they avoided gluten-containing foods. In short order, the team chef replaced wheat-based pasta with rice, oats, corn, and quinoa and expanded his culinary repertoire with dozens of gluten-free recipes. The racers initially said, "Where's the bread?" but their cravings subsided when they were served gluten-free toast with salmon caviar, baked salmon with avocado mousse, gluten-free coconut cake with sheep's milk yogurt (I love *yogurt de brebis* when I'm in France, Switzerland, or even stateside), and baked chicken curry with marinated turkey skewers and prunes.

"Unless the cyclists love what they're eating," said Garmin sports psychologist Allen Lim, "unless they can celebrate dining with one another and enjoy what they're eating, then they just won't perform. If the food is bad, they won't ride at all."

Novak Djokovic, the world's number-one tennis player, said that cutting out bread, pasta, and his father's famous pizza took him to the summit of the tennis world. (His parents owned a pizza restaurant named Red Bull in the Serbian ski resort town of Kopaonik.)

Early in his career, Djokovic (pronounced Jo-ko-vich) would hit the wall during hard-fought matches—play in listless manner, call for the trainer during changeovers, or even call it quits. "One time I collapsed and lay on my back like a beached whale," he said. TV commentators attributed his spiritless exertions to asthma, but that was guesswork.

A few years ago, a nutritionist and doctor named Igor Cetojevic watched Djokovic play Frenchman Jo-Wilfried Tsonga at the Australian Open, a Grand Slam tournament, from his home in Serbia. Although Djokovic was up two-sets-to-one, he was fading quickly under the hot sun Down Under. Djokovic had trouble breathing and asked the umpire if he could take a toilet break, where he vomited violently. When the woozy Djokovic returned, he staggered around the court and only won four games in losing the last two sets.

Dr. Cetojevic had a feeling he knew what was ailing his fellow Serb: an imbalance in his digestive system caused by gluten and a triggering of accumulating toxins in his intestines. The nutritionist reached out to the Djokovic camp and said he thought he could help Novak.

Under Dr. Cetojevic's guidance, Djokovic overhauled his diet to rid himself of excess sugar and gluten-containing foods before the start of the 2011 season. Gone were the candy bars and sugary sweets he snacked on before matches, thinking that's what he had to do to keep up his energy. Gone was the pizza and pasta, mainstays of his pre-match meals. Instead, he adopted a diet of gluten-free pasta, brown rice, and oatmeal, as well as fruit and leafy green vegetables. In 2011, Djokovic had his greatest season ever, netting three Grand Slam titles, ten tournament wins, and a fifty-three match win streak. His 2015 season has been impressive as well, capturing Wimbledon and the Australian Open. After claiming the Wimbledon crown, Djokovic knelt on the grass court, picked a bit of grass, and chewed it. "It's gluten-free," he quipped to the press afterward.

In the celebrity world, dozens of A-listers have embraced the gluten-free lifestyle, from Kim Kardashian to Miley Cyrus to Gwyneth Paltrow, who released a gluten-free cookbook entitled *It's All Good: Delicious, Easy Recipes That Will Make Your Look Good and Feel Great.* Lady Gaga has touted gluten-free as an ideal weight-loss tool, while gluten-free Chelsea Clinton made sure her wedding cake was baked without wheat or other gluten-containing grains.

It's amazing how quickly gluten-free went from an obscure term that no one has heard of to having its own section in supermarkets and health food stores. I've even stepped into specialty stores that are entirely gluten-free, and pretty much any sit-down restaurant chain worth its sea salt has gluten-free items on the menu. From Applebee's to BJ's to Chili's to Duffy's Sports Grill to East Side Mario's to Fleming's Prime Steakhouse to Godfather's Pizza...you could go through the alphabet and find restaurants with gluten-free entrees.

Gluten-free has definitely become part of the pop culture.

GUMMING UP THE WORKS

It's estimated that just 1 percent of the U.S. population cannot tolerate gluten in their diets, although I believe the number is much higher, given how our digestive systems are ill-equipped to digest wheat and similar grains. Dr. Alessio Fasano, director of the Center for Celiac Research at Massachusetts General Hospital for Children, says he figures that around 7 percent of the U.S. population has some kind of sensitivity to gluten.

"Nutritionally speaking, gluten is useless," said Dr. Fasano. "It doesn't do anything for us. Eating a lot of gluten is like asking your gastrointestinal system to do an impossible mission: to digest something that's not digestible," said the pediatric gastroenterologist.

The reason why our bodies have trouble with the gluten in wheat, rye, and barley is because most of us lack the specific enzymes to fully break down and absorb gluten. The result is that large blocks of undigested protein find their way into the small intestine, where they slow the absorption of other valuable nutrients, causing digestive stress and leading to feelings of fatigue and lack of energy.

Dr. Fasano said that the digestive systems in most people can handle these "indigestible" fragments of gluten without a hitch, but when you eliminate or cut back on gluten-bearing foods, the body can focus on other things, like carrying oxygen to the muscles. This is why some doctors theorize that eliminating gluten boosts athletic performance.

Gluten consumption will take a heavy toll if you have celiac disease, which is less common and more extreme than gluten sensitivity but still strikes around one in every 133 Americans. Celiac disease is defined as an autoimmune disorder that can occur in genetically predisposed people where the ingestion of gluten-containing foods leads to damage in the small intestine. Celiac disease is hereditary, meaning it runs in families. That's another reason I underwent the 23andMe genetic testing.

Currently, the only treatment for celiac disease or gluten intolerance is lifelong adherence to a strict gluten-free diet. I'm not the Chicken Little type who says the sky is falling and you have to join me in going gluten-free, but this is something you should pay attention to, especially if you feel bloated or don't have much energy after eating certain foods such as commercially made breads, rolls, cakes, cupcakes, churros, doughnuts, pies, and pastries. (Which you really should stay away from because these processed foods are filled with sugar and unhealthy fats.)

That said, you would be doing your body a favor by consuming fewer foods with gluten, especially if you're experiencing any of the telltale symptoms that point toward a gluten intolerance or sensitivity. You'd be in good company these days: around a quarter of U.S. adults say they are trying to reduce or completely avoid gluten in their diets, according to the marketing firm NPD Group's Dieting Monitor.

If you think you may be gluten intolerant, you will have to take one of several serologic or blood tests available that screen for celiac disease antibodies. The most common one looks like a high school algebra equation: it's called the tTG-lgA test. If test results suggest celiac disease, your doctor will likely recommend a biopsy of your small intestine to confirm the diagnosis.

As for the lesser degree of gluten sensitivity, keep in mind that any gluten sensitivity will not show up in standard blood work so you need to track your symptoms. Here are several warning signs to look for:

1. **Digestive issues.** Got gas? Feeling constipated? Dealing with diarrhea? These are the most common signs of gluten sensitivity that crop up in the digestive tract.

2. **Skin problems.** If you "break out" after eating blueberry muffins or pancakes or any other wheat product, you could have sensitivity to gluten. Rashes—marked by raised bumps on the skin—most often occur on the knees, back, elbows, buttocks, and the back of the neck. Acne and a flushed complexion are other manifestations. Two skin conditions known as *keratosis pilaris* and *dermatitis herpetiformis* have direct connections to gluten sensitivity.

3. **Feelings of exhaustion.** If you're hitting the wall like a Tour de France cyclist in the French Alps—and it's not yet noontime—gluten may be to blame. Gluten intolerance or sensitivity may interfere with natural sleep patterns, causing you to wake up feeling unrefreshed and not ready to attack the day.

4. **Migraines.** A study from Royal Hallamshire Hospital in Sheffield, United Kingdom discovered that gluten could trigger migraines and intense headaches for those who are intolerant to gluten. The patient's heightened immune responses, which were precipitated by the ingestion of gluten, was thought to be the leading factor causing the headaches. If you experience a migraine within an hour or two of eating gluten-containing foods, that's highly indicative of gluten sensitivity.

5. **Autoimmune diseases.** Gluten intolerance and/or sensitivity can be an underlying cause of diseases such as rheumatoid arthritis, Hashimoto's disease, multiple

sclerosis, and psoriasis. Joint pain and muscle aches are common symptoms of gluten intolerance.

6.   **Hormone imbalances.** Women with irregular menstrual cycles or who are having trouble getting pregnant should know that consuming gluten-containing foods may put stress on the adrenal glands, which upsets the balance of the endocrine system.

7.   **Emotional issues and mood.** If someone you love is often irritable and given to sudden, irrational mood shifts, or is anxious and depressed, then gluten could be a culprit.

8.   **Neurological symptoms.** If you're dizzy, losing your balance, experiencing patches of vertigo, or have tingly sensations in your extremities, this could be indicative of inflammation in your nervous system—inflammation that may be at least partially caused by the way your immune system responds to gluten in the digestive tract.

9.   **Family history.** It stands to reason that one of the best predictors of gluten intolerance or sensitivity is family history.

If you're experiencing several of these symptoms, try eliminating all gluten foods from your diet for two weeks to a month and see how you feel. If your symptoms show moderate to extreme improvement, I recommend continuing your gluten-free diet. Quoting the aforementioned Dr. Fasano, gluten consumption confers zero health benefits, so eliminating it from your diet and replacing gluten-containing grains with healthier alternatives can only be a good thing.

LOOKING TO THE PLANET

I really wonder if the rise in the demand for gluten-free products stems from the way we grow wheat in this country—as a monocrop that's sprayed with pesticides and then "bleached" and stripped of important nutrients during the refining process. Thank goodness there's no GMO wheat being grown, although Monsanto has developed a "transgenic" wheat called MON 71800, which is glyphosate-resistant via a CP4/maize EPSPS gene. Sounds totally natural and organic, doesn't it?

Monsanto did all the environmental risk assessments, and government regulatory agencies approved the use of this genetically modified wheat in food, but American farmers told Monsanto that they were worried about the loss of markets in Europe and Asia because these nations won't allow the importation of grains containing genetically modified wheat. So Monsanto stood down.

This is what I mean when I say that our dietary choices can aid in the healing of our planet. If all of us choose to consume less foods with gluten—particularly from wheat—then we'll see less monocrop agriculture and fewer pesticide-sprayed crops. If we can consume less gluten by cutting back on commercial pastas, breads, and sweets and substitute those grains and carbohydrates with a variety of different plant foods that can be grown using polyculture and/or permaculture principles, we're going to have a healthier planet. And you'll likely feel better than you have in a long time.

One way you can ensure that there are no detectable levels of gluten in the foods you consume is to look for the designation gluten-free on the label. You can also be proactive in your avoidance of gluten by choosing one or more of the numerous healthful substitutes for gluten-containing grains used in recipes calling for wheat, rye, or barley.

Here's a list of those gluten-free whole grains as well as nuts and legumes, which are naturally gluten-free:

- amaranth

- buckwheat

- quinoa

- canihua

- millet

- oats (make sure they're labeled as gluten-free)

- corn (look for the non-GMO variety)

- tree nuts, including almond and pecan

- legumes and beans, including black beans and garbanzo

- coconut

- brown, red, wild, and black rice

Gluten is contained in small amounts in several processed foods including sauces, salad dressings, and beverages. Gluten is also contained in many dietary supplements. To ensure the supplements you're consuming are free of gluten, make sure to look for the words "gluten-free" on the label. Gluten-free products must meet the FDA definition, which requires a food or supplement contain less than 20 parts per million of gluten and be free of any gluten-containing grains or their derivatives, unless there are processing steps involved to specifically remove the gluten.

So here's the big picture that you can keep in the back of your mind. The food industry follows demand very closely, so the less gluten we consume from gluten-containing grains, the more biodiversity we promote. I grow nostalgic, just like anyone else, when the Midwest farmlands are referred to as the "bread basket of America," but a little less cereal grains and a little more diversity in our farmlands would be an important step in healing the planet and our bodies.

For more information on gluten-free foods and supplements, visit www.PlanetHealThyself.com.

7

The Power of Plants

As an organic farmer in a mixed agriculture (polyculture) environment, we raise livestock and grow crops at the Heal the Planet Farm in Southern Missouri. I personally subscribe to what you would call an eco-friendly omnivorous diet, meaning that I consume a combo of animal and plant foods.

I'll have something to say about consciously raised animal foods in my next chapter, but for now, I want to talk up the amazing benefits of plants. Personally, I don't know what my life would be like without the incredible variety of tastes and life-sustaining health benefits that come from consuming plant foods—fruits, vegetables, nuts, seeds, legumes/beans, herbs, spices, and grains. I imagine you feel the same way, and if not, you certainly will by the end of this chapter.

Plants-based foods are as old as creation. We learn in Genesis that God said to Adam and Eve, "I will give you every seed-bearing plant on the face of the whole earth and every tree that has fruit with seed in it. They will be yours for food" (Genesis 1:29). And in case the first couple didn't catch that, God reminded Adam and Eve—after the Fall—that "you will eat the plants of the field" (Genesis 3:18b).

We receive so many marvelous nutrients from plants that grow in the earth, starting with a process known as biological transmutation, an action in which organisms in the soil take inorganic nutrients and convert them into organic substances that can be consumed by humans directly, or by animals and then by humans.

I'll never forget how Jerry Frye, a fellow farmer in Missouri, explained this to me. We were out in the fields one day, and Jerry knelt down in a pasture of mixed species of forage. He plucked several blades of grass, a few herbs, some forbs and legumes, and held them up.

"Ah, tiny solar panels, capturing the power of the sun to transfer its energy to the animals and then to us," he said, painting a wonderful word picture.

Everywhere I looked I saw green grasslands—and planted fields—utilizing the power of the sun through photosynthesis, a chemical process whereby plants capture the sun's radiant energy and use carbon dioxide and water from the environment to convert sunlight into life-sustaining nourishment. The result—live nutrients in plant foods—becomes the building blocks of nutrition and the foundation of a diet that's good for your entire body, your waistline, your future health, and the environment.

No matter how powerful the sun is, however, plants won't grow well in poor or barren soil. That's why I've talked about the importance of topsoil a great deal in *Planet Heal Thyself*, because when soil is healthy, plants thrive. Nowhere is the power of sunlight more evident than in the life of green plants. Cereal grasses, vegetables, fruits, nuts, seeds, herbs, and spices give us a broad array of vitamins, minerals, proteins, and enzymes as well as access to thousands of natural chemicals known as phytonutrients—*phyto* being the Greek word for plant.

Phytonutrients, which help protect plants from the UV rays of the sun, germs, fungi, insects, and other threats, help humans as well because of their health-promoting qualities and the way they keep our bodies working properly. There are numerous types of phytonutrients that are also known as antioxidants, the so-called "crime fighters" in your body. Antioxidants are compounds that preserve and protect cells in the body from free-radical damage.

Free radicals—the oxygen-containing molecules known for their instability and their potential to harm cells that may lead to health challenges—are something you don't want running rampant within your system. Tens of thousands of these unstable molecules are generated within the body every day; this means you really should pay attention to consuming a wide array of phytonutrients by eating fruits, veggies, herbs, spices, and seeds, all of which contain high amounts of antioxidants that can put a stop to the damaging chain of free radical formation.

Plant foods contain phytonutrients such as anthocyanins, phenolics, indoles, flavonoids, and carotenoids. These beneficial compounds help support good memory function, cardiovascular health, and a healthy weight—just to name a few of the benefits that come from consuming a wide assortment of plant foods.

Many of the vivid colors you see in fruits and vegetables—the reds, greens, oranges, purples, and yellows—are pigments with health-promoting properties. Green vegetables owe their pigment to chlorophyll. Tomatoes and watermelon are red because of a carotenoid antioxidant known as lycopene. Blueberries are colored by the phytochemical anthocyanin, which is also found in blue, black, and purple fruits such as açai berries, blackberries, and dark plums.

Pigments with health-promoting properties color every fruit and vegetable. Let's break it down by the color:

- **Purple/blue:** blueberries, blackberries, purple grapes, plums, prunes, raisins, currants, elderberry, black mission figs, eggplant, beets, and purple cabbage

- **Yellow/orange:** oranges, peaches, nectarines, papayas, pineapples, grapefruit, tangerines, mangoes, lemons, apricots, sweet potatoes, cantaloupe, carrots, yellow squash, yellow and orange peppers, pumpkin, and corn

- **Green:** salad greens, kiwi, broccoli, avocados, Brussels sprouts, chives, green onions, parsley, celery, asparagus, cilantro, green beans, spinach, peppers, Swiss chard, and kale

- **Red:** tomatoes, raspberries, apples, strawberries, pomegranates, cherries, red peppers, radishes, red onion, and watermelon

- **White:** bananas, pears, dates, peaches, coconut, potatoes, Turkish figs, jicama, cauliflower, garlic, ginger, mushrooms, onions, leeks, shallots, artichokes, and bamboo shoots

These colors have been associated with powerful health benefits:

- **Blue/purple fruits and vegetables** support urinary tract health, promote memory function, and support cellular and brain health.

- **Yellow/orange fruits and vegetables** do the heavy lifting against free radicals that roam around your body, looking for cells they can damage. Yellow/orange fruits and vegetables also support cardiovascular health and healthy inflammation levels.

- **Green fruits and vegetables** support the body's detoxification efforts and promote a healthy heart.

- **Red fruits and vegetables** support healthy inflammation levels as well as cardiovascular health.

- **White fruits and vegetables** nurture intestinal function, and support healthy blood-sugar levels and a healthy immune system.

There are dozens and dozens of powerful examples of phytonutrient-containing foods. I'm going to single out five of my favorite plant foods in each category of fruits, vegetables, nuts, seeds, legumes/beans, herbs, spices, plant-based fats, and grains. By adding these phytonutrient powerhouses to your daily diet, you are sure to experience health benefits you never knew you always wanted.

Some of these plants foods will be totally new to you, and others will be very familiar as your mother undoubtedly "encouraged" you to eat them. While each of these plant foods are healthful to the body in most any form, I recommend you consume organic versions whenever possible.

FRUITS

1. **Grapes** contain resveratrol, an antioxidant that is found in the fruit, purple grape juice, and red wine that supports healthy blood-sugar levels, supports the immune system and helps negate the effects of a calorie-laden diet. Resveratrol's cholesterol-supporting benefits make it ideal for those concerned about heart health and may help explain the "French Paradox." The French have the highest per-capita consumption of wine in the world, eat a diet loaded with butter, cheese, and cream, but they have a much lower rate of coronary heart

disease than Americans and deadly heart attacks claim half the victims in France as they do in the United States.

As I discussed in Chapter 5, there really aren't any genetically modified fruits on the market—Hawaiian papaya being the lone exception—so seedless grapes as well as watermelons and oranges do not contain GMOs. Seedless fruits are created from hybridization and are generally bred for convenience: people don't like eating or spitting out seeds. It's a source of debate whether these hybrid fruits and vegetables are as nutritious as the traditional varieties, but I always err on the side of caution. If you see some deep purple or light green organic grapes *with* seeds, then grab them and go.

2. **Pomegranate,** with 613 seeds and one of the oldest known fruits (the Old Testament refers to pomegranate as the fruit of royalty), is revered as a symbol of health, fertility, and eternal life. A great way to include pomegranates in your diet is to sprinkle pomegranate seeds onto your salad.

Pomegranates don't get taken home nearly enough from the health food store or the farmers market, however, because it's a hassle getting those seeds out—the only edible part of this red fruit. You can turn this difficult chore into a breeze by cutting off the stem, using a paring knife to cut out the crown of the pomegranate, and then cutting the fruit into sections, being careful not to cut into the seeds. Once you've broken up the pomegranate, immerse the fruit into a large bowl of cool water and let it soak for five minutes.

The seeds should separate from the membrane rather easily. You can eat pomegranate seeds out of your hand and in smoothies, but I find they are great in salads. Just be sure that when you seed a pomegranate you're wearing old clothes or an apron because a ripe and juicy pomegranate makes quite a mess.

Pomegranates contain high levels of flavonoids and polyphenols, which are potent antioxidants that support heath. When turned into a tart and tangy juice, pomegranate has more antioxidants than green tea, blueberries, and cranberries.

3.   That's not to say that **blueberries** aren't holding up their end of the nutritional bargain. Long a favorite in the Rubin household, blueberries are a big part of our smoothies as well as a topping for salads and desserts. Low in calories—just 80 per cup—and practically fat-free, blueberries are loaded with fiber that keeps you feeling full longer.

For such a small berry, this fruit sure offers huge health benefits. The antioxidant compound known as anthocyanin gives blueberries their deep blue color and supports digestive and heart health because of the way they go after free radicals. A University of Illinois at Urbana-Champaign study on the effects of blueberries on prostate health showed excellent results. Because blueberries, like cranberries, contain compounds that prevent bacteria from sticking to bladder walls, doctors say that blueberries can help support urinary tract health.

Sure, a pint of blueberries can be pricy, as I noted in a previous chapter, but blueberries should be viewed as worth their weight in gold with every single delicious bite.

4.   The vibrant red **raspberry** is a delicious high-antioxidant, high-fiber food that takes time to be digested, which means that you feel fuller longer. The insoluble fiber helps ease elimination, and the ellagic acid in raspberries is said to support cellular structure.

Ellagic acid is an antioxidant found in generous amounts in raspberries and pomegranates and to a lesser extent in strawberries, cranberries, walnuts, and pecans. This antioxidant is reputed to support healthy cellular development, retard the growth of unhealthy cells, and possess excellent benefits for female health.

5. "An apple a day keeps the doctor away" is a rhyming and pithy proverb that dates back to the Civil War. The first iteration went like this: "Eat an apple upon going to bed, and you'll keep the doctor from earning his bread."

Apples eaten any time of day are wonderful; they are also a great pre-meal snack to assuage hunger pangs. The reason is the phytonutrients in apples help you regulate your blood sugar by preventing spikes through a variety of mechanisms. Apples contain flavonoids such as quercetin, which can assist alpha-amylase and alpha-glucosidase, enzymes that break down starch and disaccharides—complex sugars—into glucose. These enzymes are involved in the breakdown of complex carbohydrates into simple sugars, so your digestion will thank you.

Apples pack a big antioxidant punch underneath the skin of Red Delicious, Golden Delicious, Gala, Fuji, Granny Smith, Braeburn, and Honeycrisp apples. (There are 7,500 varieties worldwide.) Scientists have calculated the antioxidant power in apples to equal more than 1,500 milligrams of vitamin C.

Another thing I like about apples beyond the antioxidant protection is the presence of pectin, a soluble fiber that supports blood cholesterol health by lowering levels of LDL cholesterol in the body. In a health study of about 40,000 U.S. women, researchers analyzed their apple consumption and their heart health. After controlling for other fruits along with vegetables, fiber, and other nutrients, the study found that women who ate at least one apple a day developed 22 percent fewer heart health challenges than women who ate no apples.

So maybe an apple a day really does keep the doctor away.

VEGETABLES

1.   Less than ten years ago, nobody had heard of **kale**. By "nobody," I mean the average American. You had to be really into health foods to be aware of this bitter, leafy green plant food that wasn't going to win many taste awards. For everyone else, kale was off the radar screen.

Now you see bags of kale salad, kale chips, kale cakes, and kale smoothies being offered in health food stores and kale in restaurants and delis. Parents are even naming their children after the vegetable. Hailed as a superfood and a rising superstar, kale has seen a 400 percent increase on restaurant menus since 2008. Even McDonald's—McDonald's!—is testing breakfast bowls with kale and using the popular green in salads and smoothies. What's next—kale in their Shamrock Shakes?

We'll have to see how everything pans out, but here's an interesting thought: if McDonald's adds a little kale to their salads or their smoothies, the fast-food giant becomes the number-one purchaser of kale in the U.S. That's how much of an influencer this fast-food giant can be.

Until that happens, kale—a cousin to mustard greens—is still a niche plant food, at least compared to the more common lettuces. Kale, a cruciferous vegetable that comes from the same family as cabbage, broccoli, and cauliflower, is filled with fiber—you can tell by its chewy texture. Kale also contains essential nutrients such as calcium, iron, and vitamins A, C, and K as well as antioxidants lutein and beta-carotene. One cup of kale has only 36 calories and 0 grams of fat.

Kale is a superb food that supports healthy inflammation response, upper respiratory health, the immune system, digestive health, and cardiovascular function. If kale isn't part of your salad mix, then it's time you jump aboard the kale bandwagon.

2. **Broccoli** is a lot better known to American taste buds than kale but is not universally loved. I was a freshman in high school when President G.W. Bush (41) made headlines after banning broccoli on Air Force One, saying, "I haven't liked it since I was a little kid, and my mother made me eat it. I'm president of the United States, and I'm not going to eat any more broccoli!"

Broccoli, I'm happy to report, has made a major comeback in the last twenty-five years—even at the White House. President Barack Obama told student journalists in 2013 that broccoli was his favorite food, which prompted *Tonight Show* host Jay Leno to ask the President if he could put his hand on the Bible and swear allegiance to the healthy crucifer.

"Let me say this," the President responded. "I have broccoli a lot."

The *Tonight Show* audience chuckled, but this fibrous vegetable still doesn't get much respect.

Eating sprigs of uncooked broccoli in salads is a good option, although eating raw broccoli could be irritable to your digestive tract and cause gas and bloating. Because boiling broccoli in water shows the biggest losses of nutrients, you're going to be better off steaming or stir-frying broccoli, which has shown no significant loss of nutrients such as vitamin C, potassium, B_6, and vitamin A. Steaming or stir-frying also ensures that the broccoli doesn't become soft and mushy.

Broccoli's phytonutrients are impressive: sulforaphane, indole-3 carbinol, isothiocyanate, glucobrassicin; carotenoids such as zeaxanthin and beta-carotene; and a flavonoid called kaempferol. With a reputation for being high in iron, broccoli also contains some magnesium, phosphorous, and zinc and is known for its ability to aid the body in detoxification.

Now if I were president of the United States for a day, I'd declare National Broccoli Day.

3. **Beets** are another vegetable that's greeted with upturned noses at the dinner table. Though sugar beets are often genetically modified, the red roots of organic beets contain powerful phytonutrients.

You might turn into a beet lover when you hear about some of the health properties of beets. Beets contain high amounts of boron, which is directly related to the production of human sex hormones. Beets are high in many of the same vitamins and minerals as broccoli—vitamins A, B, and C, plus beta-carotene—but they're unusual in that they work to purify blood, which supports cellular structure. Beets can boost mental health because they contain two substances, betaine and tryptophan. The former substance is useful in supporting mental health, and the latter phytonutrient is known for creating a sense of relaxation and well-being.

Beets may get a bad rap for not tasting that great, but small pieces of raw beets are a delicious addition to any salad and certainly worthy of being included in a smoothie or homemade vegetable juice. Keep in mind that beets have the highest sugar content of all vegetables, which explains why sugar beets are the second largest source of sugar after sugar cane.

4. Who doesn't like **carrots**? If you live a normal life expectancy, you'll eat 10,866 carrots in your lifetime, according to Nick Watts, the producer of *The Human Footprint*, a BBC show in England.

As Bugs Bunny would say while chewing a carrot, "Eh...what's up, Doc?" Well, there's a lot up with carrots, starting with how they were originally grown as medicine, not food. According to the virtual World Carrot Museum, in A.D. 70 Greek physician Pedanius Dioscorides catalogued their possible medicinal uses during his travels as a Roman Army doctor.

Today, carrots are a popular snack and routinely tossed into soups and stews. One medium-sized carrot provides 210 percent of the average recommended amount of vitamin A as beta-carotene. Carrots are a great source of carotenoids, including beta-carotene, and they're also a surprisingly good source of calcium.

If you're thinking that carrot and carotene sound alike, there's a reason for that. A German pharmacist, Heinrich Wackenroder, discovered carotene in 1826 after he crystallized the compounds from carrot roots. The high vitamin A content, which is what carrots are known for, comes from beta-carotene, which is converted into vitamin A by the liver.

Researchers at the U.S. Department of Agriculture found that study participants who consumed two carrots per day were able to lower their cholesterol levels about 20 percent due to a soluble fiber/mineral compound called calcium pectate.

You don't have to shop for the same old orange carrots. Farmers markets are great places to find organic purple, white, red, and yellow carrots.

5. The last vegetable on my top five list is **watercress**. I can see the head scratching going on. *I've heard of watercress, Jordan, but what is it?*

Watercress is a peppery-flavored, fast-growing leafy vegetable that grows in streams and rivers. In fact, we have a small river on our Beyond Organic ranch, and one of the fun chores is taking several kids with me and gathering up huge bunches of watercress out of the water, consuming it back on the ranch, and feeding what's left over to our chickens.

Watercress features small, oval, deep green leaves with high moisture content, as you'd expect for a plant that grows in water. The leaves have a very strong, peppery aftertaste like mustard greens. Watercress is best when mixed with Romaine lettuce or fresh spinach, or added into soups. If you've ever had high tea in England, then you were likely served watercress sandwiches.

Here's something that caught my eye about watercress. Researchers at William Patterson University in New Jersey, in a study published in a Centers for Disease Control journal, listed forty-one "powerhouse fruits and vegetables," ranked by amounts of seventeen critical nutrients found in each food. A little drumbeat, please...and watercress was number one with a score of one hundred! The next five in this elite category were Chinese cabbage, chard, beet greens, spinach, and chicory.

Vitamin K, which plays an important role in blood clotting, building strong bones, and supporting a healthy heart, is the most prominent nutrient in watercress with 312 percent of the recommended value. Watercress also contains high amounts of vitamin C and vitamin A in the form of beta-carotene as well as zeaxanthin and lutein.

NUTS

1.   **Almonds** are the king of nuts and a personal favorite of mine. One of those perfect snack foods, almonds are higher in fiber than all other nuts and contain 50 percent more total fiber than peanuts as well as healthy omega-9 oleic fatty acids. Just one ounce contains one-eighth of our necessary daily protein as well as being a strong source of vitamin E, copper, and magnesium. Various medical studies show that almonds can lower cholesterol levels, support cardiovascular health, and possibly cut the risk of certain cancers.

2.   **Pecans** contain more antioxidants than any other nut, according to research from the U.S. Department of Agriculture, which is why they're high on my list. A handful of pecans contains vitamin E, calcium, magnesium, zinc, and fiber. These buttery-tasting nuts are filling and provide an important part of the Dietary Approaches to Stop Hypertension (DASH) eating plan created by the National Institutes of Health as a way to lower blood pressure.

Pecans, which make great toppings for any salad, are a rich source of oleic acid, which was found in laboratory tests conducted by researchers from Northwestern University in Chicago to have the ability to suppress certain gene activity in cells thought to trigger breast cancer. The type of vitamin E in pecans is believed to support prostate health, according to a study from Purdue University.

3. Delectable **macadamia nuts**, grown in tropical climates such as Hawaii, have a crunchy texture that makes them a delight to consume. Macadamia nuts are a superb source of vitamin A, iron, protein, thiamin, riboflavin, and folate.

Macadamia nuts contain large amounts of monosaturated fat that's known to help lower cholesterol and decrease the risk of heart disease and stroke. They are also high in calories compared to other nuts, but their high fiber and low carbohydrates more than make up the difference.

4. Rich in monosaturated fats and high in calories similar to macadamia nuts, **Brazil nuts** are known for being high in selenium, an important trace mineral. Selenium helps the body by making special proteins, called antioxidant enzymes, that play a role in preventing cell damage. Brazil nuts have about 2,500 times as much selenium as any other nut.

Brazil nuts come, as you would expect, from South American countries such as (naturally) Brazil, as well as Peru, Columbia, and Venezuela. They're found in many "mixed nut" blends sold everywhere.

5. **Walnuts** are high in protein, omega-3 fatty acids, trace minerals, and lecithin. The antioxidants in walnuts help protect against the symptoms of advanced aging and support cardiovascular and neurological health. Walnuts have shown an ability to quench free radicals.

SEEDS

1. **Chia seeds** are small edible seeds that grow abundantly in warm climates such as southern Mexico, South America, and Australia. Packed full of fiber and healthy fats such as omega-3 fatty acids, chia's fiber-rich seeds have the highest percentage of omega-3 alpha-linolenic acid (ALA) of any plant. You'll also find plenty of calcium, phosphorus, manganese, potassium, and antioxidants in chia seeds, which help support healthy blood-sugar levels and cardiovascular health and provide fiber for satiety and healthy weight management.

Chia seeds, when hydrated, swell seven to nine times their size inside the stomach and go to work inside the intestinal tract. Sprinkling chia seeds into smoothies (something I do every morning) or on salads, in cereal, baked goods, or yogurt is a good way to get these seeds into your diet.

2. **Pumpkin seeds** are usually thrown away after carving a Halloween pumpkin, but these flat, green seeds are highly nutritious and flavorful. Pumpkin seeds are especially rich in omega-3, omega-6, and omega-9 fatty acids as well as beta-sitosterol, which supports HDL cholesterol in the blood. The consumption of these seeds supports healthy prostate function in addition to providing carotenoids, iron, zinc, manganese, magnesium, phosphorus, copper, and potassium.

3. **Hemp seeds** are rich in omega-3 and omega-6 fatty acids. They are also an excellent source of gamma-linolenic acid (GLA) and contain the highest percentage of protein of any seed or grain. No other single plant source has each of the essential amino acids in such an easily digestible form.

4. **Sunflower seeds,** which promote healthy digestion and weight management, are packed with vitamins, including vitamin B_1 and B_5, vitamin E and folate, and provide important minerals such as copper,

magnesium, selenium, and phosphorous. Sunflower seeds are nature's gift from the beautiful sunflower and its rays of petals branching out from a bright yellow, seed-studded center.

There are folklore stories about Russian soldiers who were given around a cup of sunflower seeds each day as their food allotment, and they were able to live for days and weeks on nothing but sunflower seeds. In modern times, major league baseball players—especially those seeking to break a chewing tobacco habit—dig out handfuls of sunflower seeds from their back pockets, popping them into their mouths and spitting the shells into the breeze. That's sure a lot better than chewing tobacco, which likely took the life of baseball's Tony Gywnn, the hitting maestro who died in 2014 from salivary gland cancer.

5. **Flaxseeds** are an excellent source of soluble and insoluble fiber as well as omega-3 fatty acids. You'll find eight vitamins, four macrominerals, four trace minerals, and ten amino acids in flaxseeds.

Flaxseeds are a wonderful source of powerful phytonutrients, as well as mucilaginous fiber, which lubricates the bowel and promotes healthy cellular structure.

LEGUMES/BEANS

1. A lot of people don't know much about **garbanzo beans,** and some aren't even aware that they're also called chickpeas and usually mashed into the hummus you purchase in health food stores. Many people also don't know that garbanzo beans, a nutty-flavored bean indigenous to India, are the most consumed legume in the world.

Garbanzo beans are packed with magnesium, potassium, and iron. A half-cup has 5 grams of fiber and 6 grams of muscle-building protein. If you're dealing with constipation, garbanzo beans are a great way to break the logjam. A 2008 study in *Journal of the American Dietetic*

Association showed that the additional fiber in garbanzo beans helped increase the frequency of bowel movements to once daily and speed up the passage of stool through the colon.

2. **Fava beans** are not well known and are often confused with edamame because both are green-colored legumes that come in their own pod. High in protein and dietary fiber but very low in fat, fava beans may offer cardiovascular benefits and help in weight management because they slow down digestion and make you feel full longer.

Also known as broad beans, fava beans can be eaten canned, fresh, or dried. Their flavor is sweeter and richer than other beans, which makes them easier to include as a side dish. But fava beans should be soaked in water for at least six to eight hours before boiling them in water. Fava bean fans add them to salads, soups, stews, and casseroles.

What stands out to me about fava beans is how they are rich in L-dopa, an amino acid that increases dopamine levels, which is converted by the body into neurotransmitters—the brain chemicals that communicate information between the brain and our bodies. Dopamine is a special neurotransmitter that helps with focus and staying on task and supports the brain's ability to remember things.

3. Here's another legume with a reputation of helping people lose weight—**adzuki beans**. Native to East Asia and the Himalayas, adzuki beans can be used to make a form of natto, which is usually made from soaked and fermented soybeans. When adzuki beans—generally red—are boiled and mashed into a bean paste, they have a sweetness that can used as a topping for desserts or as a savory addition to main course dishes.

Adzuki beans have a high concentration of soluble fiber, so they are ideal for stabilizing cholesterol levels and assist the body in eliminating toxins.

4. **Cacao beans** have three hundred healthful compounds, such as potassium and copper, that support cardiovascular health and iron, which supports oxygen utilization throughout the body. Polyphenol compounds such as catechins, anthocyanins, and proanthocyanidins serve as antioxidants and inhibit blood platelets from forming a clot.

Cacao beans are used to make chocolate, of course, but commercially made chocolate—with added white sugar, emulsifiers, and other unhealthy ingredients—is not a health food. Healthy dark chocolate that's at least 70 percent cacao and made with organic ingredients can be a healthy treat. Even better are raw cocoa nibs that are essentially raw chocolate.

5. My last recommendation is **coffee beans**. While I'm not a coffee drinker, the bean behind the world's most popular beverage is loaded with phytonutrients. Green coffee beans (actually seeds) are coffee beans that haven't been roasted.

Roasting coffee beans reduces the amount of chlorogenic acid, a phytonutrient in coffee beans that's touted for reducing blood-sugar levels, supporting brain health and boosting metabolism, which promotes healthy weight loss.

HERBS

1. **Ashwagandha**, an Eastern Indian herb whose name comes from the Sanskrit language, is a combination of *ashva*, meaning horse, and *gandha*, meaning smell. Put them together, and you have a root with a strong horse-like smell.

Ashwagandha is considered an adaptogenic herb that supports multiple functions and systems of the body to resist many stressors of life. Described as "Indian ginseng," this herb is used by practitioners of traditional Ayurvedic medicine in India for arthritis, anxiety, insomnia, bronchitis, and fibromyalgia, but it's only been in the last couple of years that there's been a flurry of scientific studies on this herb, which is being promoted as a quintessential adaptogen.

Fifty different studies were released in 2012 and 2013, including one from Louisiana State researchers finding that ashwagandha inhibited unhealthy cell growth as well as a study from Baylor University showing that ashwagandha reduced inflammation related to type 1 diabetes.

2. **Holy basil** comes from leaves that are members of the mint family and is closely related to sweet basil. Revered in its native India as the "Queen of Herbs" and frequently grown around Hindu temples, holy basil is a powerful antioxidant with antibacterial, antifungal, and anti-inflammatory properties. Its leaves and stems contain chemical compounds such as saponins, flavonoids, triterpenoids, and tannins.

Scientific studies in the last decade have focused on its therapeutic potential for cancer patients who've undergone radiation therapy and for its stabilizing effects on diabetes sufferers. The most compelling data suggests that holy basil shows its greatest potential for those seeking to reduce stress in their lives.

3. **Aloe vera** is a plant with thick, triangular leaves that grows in dry climates. The gel inside aloe leaves is used in a myriad of skin care products and beverages as well as dietary supplements. Aloe vera gel contains high levels of vitamins, A, C, and E as well as vitamin B_{12} and folate. Aloe vera contains twenty amino acids, including seven out of the eight essential amino acids.

Though aloe vera often works great for sunburned skin, you might want to check out aloe vera juice for its antioxidants that fight free radicals found in our bodies. Its anti-inflammatory properties can help with swollen, stiff, or painful joints and is widely recommend as a digestive health tonic.

4. **Green tea** is a marvelous herb and one of the most studied and exciting botanicals today. And just what makes tea so special? The

secret behind tea lies in its high content of health-promoting agents collectively known as polyphenols or flavonoids—specifically the group known as catechins.

Green tea is the most popular form of tea around the world, mainly because it's the beverage of choice in Asia. With half the caffeine of black tea, green tea contains healthy antioxidants including epigallocatechin gallate, or EGCG, which supports the flow of blood through the vessels and is good for cardiovascular health. EGCG is a powerful antioxidant or "anti-rust" agent that supports immune system health.

I love drinking green tea but not the kind that comes in teabags, which most Americans prefer. I prefer making tea in a loose-leaf form, but not as an *infusion*, which is the way tea is often made in Europe and Asia. With an infusion, boiling water is poured over the tea leaves, herbs, and even bits of flowers and allowed to steep for three to five minutes before it's strained through a filter and into a cup.

I prefer to prepare my tea as a mixed *decoction*, which is different from an infusion in that tea leaves are mixed with bark, roots, and seeds and placed into a pot of water for five or ten minutes to soak before being set on a stove and brought to a slow boil, then allowed to simmer for ten to thirty minutes or even longer. I've found that a decoction is a better way to liberate phytonutrients from leaves as well as the more woody or fibrous spices and barks I like to combine with my tea, such as turmeric, ginger, and cinnamon. Once the decoction is fully prepared, I pour it through a strainer and into a cup. I call this process "thermal liberation" because of the way the phytonutrients are freed up through the long heating (thermal) process.

Several times per day, I'll take some reishi mushrooms that we grow in Central California and combine that with green tea in a decoction. On certain days, I'll make a decoction to support the immune and lymphatic systems that's made up of Echinacea, ashwagandha, astragalus, and milk thistle. I love the ancient art of liberating phytonutrients from these herbs and spices.

5. **Astragalus** has been used in traditional Chinese medicine for centuries as a restorative tonic. Actually a type of legume, this herb is said to offer health benefits for various conditions, including immune system support and heart health benefits. Its antioxidant effects inhibit free-radical production. Astragalus is also said to stimulate the spleen, liver, lungs, and circulatory and urinary systems.

SPICES

1. **Turmeric,** which comes from a perennial plant, is a cousin of ginger and a pungent Indian spice that imparts a vivid yellow color. Turmeric has gained significant popularity as a powerful source of antioxidants and is the ingredient in mustard that gives the condiment its famous yellow color.

Turmeric provides the foundational benefits of healthy metabolism, digestion, and healthy immune system function in the body while supporting healthy joint function and youthful skin by providing antioxidants that support your cells against oxidative stress due to free radicals. Turmeric also supports cardiovascular health.

I like to make a decoction using turmeric and other powerful spices. Each day, I take two tablespoons of dried turmeric, one tablespoon of ginger, one tablespoon of cinnamon, and one tablespoon of clove to my tea and essentially let this simmer for hours. I drink this decoction a few times a day, mixing it with lemon juice and coconut cream as the added fat helps to deliver the curcumin contained in turmeric.

2. **Ginger** is a pungent spice that comes from the underground stem of the *Zingiber officinale* plant often found in South America, India, China, Mexico, and several other countries. Each variety of

ginger possesses its own distinctive flavor and aroma, and all you have to do is lean down toward a cutting board and take in a whiff of its sweet perfumed sharpness to encounter one of the most unique sensory experiences you'll ever come across. The special flavor of ginger adds bite to Asian dishes as well as to vegetable sides.

Ginger has a historical tradition of promoting gastrointestinal health and supporting numerous systems of the body, including fighting occasional nausea. Ginger also contains chemicals that inhibit toxic bacteria in the digestive tract while it promotes friendly bacteria, which is why this spice is effective in conditions such as constipation and diarrhea. Ginger reduces the total volume of gastric juices, stimulates fat-digesting bile, and restores balance to proper digestive function. In addition, ginger contains potent compounds called *gingerols*, which support healthy inflammation response and promote healthy joints, ligaments and tendons.

There's a lot to like about the world's most cultivated spice.

3. **Cinnamon** is a fragrant spice that's been used since biblical times for its health and culinary properties. The Romans used cinnamon to take the edge off their strong, bitter wine, and the Greeks used it to season their meat and vegetables. The exotic, sweet-flavored spice comes from the outer brown bark of *Cinnamomum* trees.

Research has shown that cinnamon may lower blood sugar in people with diabetes, reduce inflammation, fight bacteria, and provide antioxidant effects. A little bit of cinnamon goes a long way: one teaspoon of cinnamon packs as much antioxidant power as a half cup of blueberries.

I find cinnamon to be absolutely amazing and love the sweet aroma and health benefits it brings to my daily decoctions. You might want to consider having an infusion or decoction of cinnamon, especially after eating a high-sugar meal, because cinnamon, as well as turmeric, can help curb the negative effects of eating such foods.

According to Penn State researchers, overweight men who ate a plate full of chicken with sauce, Italian herb bread, and a biscuit saw their triglycerides levels shoot way up, which raised the risk of heart disease. When cinnamon and turmeric were consumed, however, the triglyceride response dropped by 30 percent, which is not too shabby.

4. **Cloves** are the dried, unopened pink flower buds of the evergreen tree, and I love adding a tablespoon of clove to my decoction. These tiny buds are giants when it comes to their anti-fungal, antibacterial, antiseptic, and analgesic qualities. Cloves are packed with antioxidants and are good sources of omega-3 fatty acids, fiber, vitamins, and minerals like manganese.

Clove has been used for years to help with upset stomachs, and clove oil—an essential oil—is used for diarrhea and intestinal gas. The component responsible for clove's powerful effects as well as pungent smell is eugenol, which has been shown to be effective in establishing an environment in the digestive tract that's unfriendly to harmful organisms.

5. How could I not include **garlic** in my list? Although when it comes to garlic, I nearly blew it when I was courting my future wife, Nicki. At the time, I was doing a juice cleanse and adding nine cloves of raw garlic to the mix. I didn't think anything of it, but Nicki sure got a whiff when I pulled her close during a slow dance at a friend's wedding!

Garlic, an herb that's widely used as a flavoring in cooking, has been used for thousands of years as a natural remedy to prevent and treat a wide range of conditions and diseases. Hippocrates, the "father of Western medicine," declared garlic to be an ideal food and prescribed garlic for a variety of ailments 2,500 years ago. The original

Olympic athletes in Greece relied on garlic as their PES—performance-enhancing spice of choice.

Garlic has been studied extensively for its health benefits. A 2001 study published in the journal *Advances in Therapy* found that a garlic supplement can reduce the number of colds by 63 percent, which perhaps explains why, back in the day, people used to wear necklaces of garlic to ward off germs and vampires.

Garlic has been shown to support the lowering of blood pressure, even when compared to prescription drugs. By lowering LDL cholesterol, garlic can help decrease the risk of heart disease. Physical performance is enhanced as well, which is why those Greek Olympians were on to something many centuries ago.

A 2005 study published in the *Indian Journal of Physiology and Pharmacology* found participants with heart disease who took garlic oil for six weeks saw a reduction in peak heart rate by 12 percent. This was accompanied by an improvement in their physical endurance during treadmill exercise.

PLANT-BASED FATS

1. One of the first solid foods we introduced to our son, Joshua, was fresh, organic Florida **avocado**, which has an abundance of healthy monounsaturated fats, vitamin E, and fiber.

I'm a huge avocado fan. With their creamy, rich texture and plenty of protein and enzymes galore, especially the fat-digesting enzyme lipase, if my salad doesn't have avocado, I feel like something is missing. It's a good idea to include avocado in your salads because researchers found that adding avocado to a mixed salad increased the absorption of carotenoids in leafy greens and carrots by two to six times. Avocados also contain two phytochemicals, lutein and zeaxanthin, that are essential to eye health.

2. Similar to avocados, **olives** are rich in monosaturated fats that support healthy cholesterol levels and cardiovascular health. Olives are a rich source of omega-9 fatty acids, an unsaturated fatty acid known to support healthy blood-sugar levels.

Olives can provide a zesty addition to any salad, but most people consume the oil of the olive more often. Olive oil is best consumed on food and unheated. Look for certified organic extra-virgin olive oil in a dark bottle since light coming into clear bottles can decrease some of the important health properties of the oil as well as its freshness. Extra-virgin olive oil is produced from the first cold pressing of the olives, and that's where you'll get the most antioxidants and other nutrients. Choose a colorful oil with a rich aroma.

Olives and olive oil offer a diverse range of antioxidants and phytonutrients, including a phenol known as hydroxytyrosol, called the most powerful antioxidant to date according to its ORAC value, or Oxygen Radical Absorbance Capacity, referring to its ability to absorb cell-damaging free radicals.

3. **Coconut** is neither a fruit nor a vegetable, but is classified as a fibrous, one-seeded drupe. The coconut meat is off-the-charts high in dietary fiber—four times as much fiber as oat bran and twice as much fiber as wheat bran or flaxseed. You can easily add coconut to beverages, smoothies, and juices.

The trifecta of coconut, coconut water, and coconut oil have earned reputations as superfoods and are among the top-selling products in health food stores today. What often gets overlooked is the energy-boosting fat that comes from coconut. Coconut is not only a healthy source of fiber, but it also contains healthy fats known as MCFAs (medium-chain fatty acids). Coconut has a small amount of high-quality protein, but combined with healthy fats and fiber, coconut is a superstar food on any list. Both the fiber and the good fats in coconut are helpful in cleansing the body and help promote a positive intestinal environment.

One of my go-to ingredients every time I make a smoothie is raw coconut cream, which can do a clean-up number on stored toxins, acting much like a powerful solvent to leave your body's insides as clean as a top. The saturated fat contained in coconut cream is a healthy high-energy source that your body can easily metabolize and turn into quick energy, all done without raising your blood cholesterol level or adding pounds to your frame.

4. While coconut is getting all the love today, I want to also call your attention to **palm oil**, which is rich in tocotrienols, an antioxidant form of vitamin E said to support cellular health and promote a healthy cardiovascular system. Palm oil is a stable cooking fat that resists going rancid. Because this oil solidifies at room temperature, you can use it in baking.

5. Ever heard of an herb called **sea buckthorn**? You probably haven't, but the leaves, flowers, and fruits of this herb, when pressed into oil, are used to make a natural remedy used to treat ailments ranging from arthritis to gout to skin rashes. Sea buckthorn oil is probably best known for promoting healthy skin aiding in the healing of burns, sores, wounds, and eczema.

GRAINS

1. Five, six years ago, nobody had heard of quinoa (pronounced *keen-wah*), but this fast-rising non-gluten grain (technically a seed) is riding a huge wave of popularity.

Quinoa grows in the Andes Mountains of South America, although it's now being cultivated in Colorado's high-elevation San Luis Valley at 7,500 feet. Recently, I began consuming **black quinoa**, which I believe even tops white quinoa, the version more widely available in stores. Black quinoa, which is a bit earthier than white quinoa, keeps its striking dark color even after it's been cooked.

When it comes to any sort of grain, the darker it is, the better, which is why in this section you'll notice that all five grains have rich, dark colors. Black quinoa has a slightly nutty flavor and a crunchier texture than white quinoa, its exotic black color coming from anthocyanins that help protect the body against free radicals and supports heart and cellular health.

Black quinoa is a complete protein, so you'll find all the amino acids required by the body. High in fiber as well as manganese and magnesium, black quinoa contains large amounts of two flavonoids, quercetin and kaempferol, that have been shown to have anti-inflammatory and anti-viral qualities in animal studies.

2. I doubt you've heard of my next grain—**cañihua**, which also deserves a pronunciation guide. (Cañihua is pronounced *ka-ni-wah*, and on some websites, it's spelled kaniwa.)

What is cañihua? Well, you could call cañihua the little cousin of quinoa because it also grows in the Andean highlands and has a similar nutritional profile. Cañihua is only grown in Peru and Bolivia, and exports are minimal, so you will probably have to go to the Internet to purchase from an online retailer, although my guess is that health food stores will soon begin carrying this brilliant red-colored grain.

The extra effort will be worth it because little-known cañihua punches above its weight, as they say, and has even more flavonoids than quinoa.

3. Another non-gluten grain I like a lot is millet, which usually comes in a golden color. Once again, I've found a colored version I prefer—**purple**.

Purple millet, like its golden cousin, is one of the most digestible and non-allergenic grains available and is great for digestive health because of the way it hydrates your colon and feeds the microflora in your gut. Purple millet also shows high antioxidant activity, and the vitamin B$_3$ (niacin) supports healthy cholesterol levels.

4. Staying with the theme of this section, my next grain is **black rice**, which is even better than brown rice, which everyone knows is better than white rice.

Black rice offers far superior health benefits to brown rice; because of its dark color, black rice packs a greater antioxidant punch containing anthocyanins—the same phytonutrients found in blueberries and blackberries.

Back in ancient times, Chinese emperors kept black rice all to themselves, which is why it's called the "forbidden rice" in Chinese folklore. Low in calories, low in glucose content, and rich in fiber and iron, black rice would make a great addition to your pantry.

5. Everyone loves corn, and I do, too—the non-GMO kind. But have you tried **purple corn**? I have, and I love this corn that comes from the Andes Mountains in Peru, as does quinoa and cañihua. The purplish color comes from anthocyanins, a complex flavonoid that produces blue, red, and purple colors in our foods. These anthocyanins have anti-inflammatory properties and encourage regeneration of the tissues.

Purple corn is *really* purple; I encourage you to go online and check out photos. An extraordinarily healthful food, purple corn looks like it's painted. The taste is succulent with a bit of a fruity flavor. But the ORAC value is a chart topper with a score of 10,800 (per 100 grams), a number that far outranks any other corn variety and is more than double what blueberries offer (4,669 per 100 grams).

Purple in any fruit or vegetable is very popular these days and a good sign that the produce contains higher-than-usual beneficial phytonutrients.

A CLOSING THOUGHT

While I don't want to say that consuming an exclusively plant-based diet is a better way to heal the planet, what I will say in no uncertain terms is that consuming organic, non-GMO, heirloom grown fruits, vegetables, grains, seeds, and legumes absolutely promotes polyculture and permaculture diversity, which ultimately provides healing to the planet and its people.

If we were to consume a wide variety of plant foods every day, the massive infrastructure of monocrop agriculture would be largely destroyed. That would be a great thing for the planet because when you replace monocrop agriculture with polyculture or permaculture, proper crop rotation and rebuilding the soil will really make a positive difference in the health of our planet.

For more information on the most powerful plant foods on the planet, including phytonutrient-rich fruits, vegetables, nuts, seeds, legumes, grains, and nutritional supplements, visit www.PlanetHealThyself.com.

8

Avoid Eight Common Allergens

DID YOU KNOW THAT FOOD MANUFACTURERS ARE REQUIRED TO LIST any of the eight common ingredients that trigger food allergies on their packaging?

Right under the listing of *Ingredients*, food manufacturers must prominently list the allergens with an advisory that says, for example, "Contains Peanuts" or "Contains Eggs." These eight, which I call the "Allergen Eight," account for an estimated 90 percent of allergic reactions to food. The eight foods are:

- milk

- eggs

- peanuts

- tree nuts (such as almonds, cashews, and walnuts)

- fish (such as salmon, tuna, and halibut)

- shellfish (such as crab, lobster, and shrimp)

- soy

- wheat

If you just glanced at that list and said to yourself, *I'm not allergic to any of those foods*, don't skip this chapter. You may not go into anaphylactic shock when you grab a handful of peanuts at the baseball game, but oftentimes there are delayed allergies and sensitivities that are difficult to pinpoint without further diagnostic testing. You should also pay close attention if you have nagging health problems that come and go or feel worse after eating certain foods because food allergies are nothing to brush off. They are a serious medical condition affecting up to 15 million Americans, including one in every thirteen children.

A food allergy results when the immune system—which is tasked with identifying and destroying germs such as bacteria and viruses—mistakenly targets a harmless food protein (known as an allergen) as a threat and attacks it. Reactions can affect the skin, the gastrointestinal tract, the respiratory tract, and in the most serious cases, the cardiovascular system.

Even if you've never experienced allergic reactions to any of these eight common foods, I think you should do your best to identify these common allergens in your diet and consider lowering the amounts you consume, finding suitable alternatives or eliminating the sources altogether.

For the rest of the chapter, I will take you on a guided tour of the top allergy-causing foods with a goal to arm you with information that can help you make informed choices when it comes to the Allergen Eight.

1. MILK

Cow's milk is the most common food allergy among infants and young children. Symptoms range from a mild reaction, such as hives, to something as severe as anaphylaxis, which threatens breathing and blood circulation.

Like everyone, I never understood *why* so many people were allergic to cow's milk; I just thought they were born that way. My consciousness was raised, however, when I visited a Pennsylvania dairy while on a speaking tour. This happened about ten years ago.

The owner insisted I sample some of his dairy products, including his grass-fed raw milk ice cream, which I found to be otherworldly. One thing I noticed is how these dairy products were easy to digest, more so than other cow's milk products I'd consumed in the past.

The dairy farmer and I got into a discussion about the makeup of cow's milk, which consists of fat, protein, carbohydrates, vitamins, minerals, and water. Cow's milk is primarily made up of two major proteins: the first is called casein (making up approximately 80 percent of the total dairy protein) and the other is lactalbumin or whey (making up the remaining 20 percent). Within the casein is a particular protein called beta-casein with two primary variants—A1 and A2—depending on the genetic makeup of the cow the milk came from.

The A1 beta-casein affects the body differently than A2 beta-casein does. Upon digestion of A1 beta-casein, a peptide—a small chain of proteins—is formed. Known as beta-casomorphin 7, or BCM7, this peptide can cause the body problems and is one reason (along with lactose intolerance) why some people complain of bloating, cramps, gas, and diarrhea after consuming dairy products made from cow's milk. What was previously understood to be symptoms of lactose intolerance may in fact be an intolerance to the A1 beta-casein protein.

This was the first time I heard of the presence of A1 beta-casein in most cow's milk—even raw, grass-fed. Could this be the reason why many can't tolerate it?

I did my own research and found that 99.9 percent of cow's milk in the U.S. contains A1 beta-casein. But outside the United States, cows in Africa, India, and the Middle East produce milk that is free of A1 beta-casein due to the fact that their cattle originated from a different species and the milk has a genetic makeup containing primarily the A2 beta-casein protein. This is why U.S. immigrants from these continents and regions say that American milk makes them feel sick.

When I started my organic farming adventure, I knew I wanted cows that produced milk with A2 beta-casein protein and were free of A1 beta-casein. I can personally attest how wonderful this milk has been for me and my family as well as thousands of family who have benefited from our "beyond organic" dairy products.

Dairy products produced from cows that produce exclusively A2 beta-casein isn't easy to find in the U.S., but hopefully that will change in the next several years. In the meantime, I suggest you do an online search and learn what you can about this important health topic.

While you're doing so, make sure to check out the work of Keith Woodford, a professor of farm management and agribusiness at New Zealand's Lincoln University who wrote the 2007 book *Devil in the Milk: Illness, Health, and the Politics of A1 and A2 Milk.* In the meantime, I recommend the consumption of dairy products made from goat's milk and sheep's milk, which *do not* contain the A2 beta-casein protein, or cow's milk that's free of A2 beta-casein.

I also believe pasture-raised cattle will produce milk less likely to cause allergic reactions as the cattle are consuming the diet that best suits them. Many individuals who are sensitive to pasteurized, homogenized cow's milk can tolerate unpasteurized or raw dairy. When consuming raw dairy, I highly recommend purchasing from a grade A dairy or at the very least from a farm that uses proper sanitization systems as there are risks from consuming dairy produced without the proper cleaning steps. Another way to reduce the incidence of allergy is to culture or ferment dairy. The fermentation process pre-digests the milk, making the proteins smaller in size and easier to digest.

Finally, here's another reason I recommend avoiding conventional milk. Not only are you potentially getting traces of bovine growth hormone, which is a genetically modified substance that is given to dairy cows to help them produce more milk, in addition consuming conventional milk products exposes you to residues of antibiotics used widely in conventional agriculture. Dairy cows are often dosed up with antibiotics and hormones, and they eat grain laced with GMOs. To me, that's a recipe for disaster.

To sum up: if you want to reduce your risk of allergic reactions or delayed sensitivities to cow's milk, consider the following:

- Seek out goat's milk, sheep's milk, and A1 beta-casein-free cow's milk.

- If consuming cow's milk, find dairy from grass-fed cows. A clean, unpasteurized source can be tolerable for many sensitive people.

- Consume sources of cultured dairy in the form of yogurt, kefir, or Amasai.

These are some of the ways to reduce dairy allergies without completely eliminating dairy, but those with suspected allergies to any and all milk should stop consuming dairy. Until you do so, you'll never be truly healthy.

2. EGGS

This is a tough one because we raise chickens on our farm, and I consume loads of pasture-raised eggs. I believe part of the issue with the allergy incidence of eggs is the way that the chickens are raised and some of the other elements that are a part of modern egg production.

There are ways to consume eggs in a healthier form, and that would be raising your own laying hens—I know, easier said than done—or shopping for pasture-raised eggs. But wait a minute. What do those phrases on egg cartons mean—"cage-free," "free-range," or "organic"? How are they different from "pasture-raised" eggs?

So far, the U.S. Department of Agriculture doesn't have a formal definition or standards for pasture-raised eggs, but what it's generally understood to mean is that regenerative farmers such as myself are raising our chickens outdoors…in the pasture with plenty of space to roam. The chickens forage their natural diet, which means pecking for insects, worms, seeds, and green plants.

That's different from free-range eggs, which means, according to USDA regulations, that the chickens have "access" to the outside. There's a reason why *access* has quote marks and it's because that's all it means. "Access" to the outside doesn't mean that the chickens *ever go* outside. Far from it.

What free-range generally means, in practical terms for large commercial egg producers, is that the chickens are not in traditional cages and are free to walk around. In actuality, though, thousands of chickens are crammed into a large warehouse with a small doggy-type door at one end of the building that opens to a small patch of dirt. Most chickens don't know the door is there—they don't read their email—so they don't avail themselves of fresh air. Instead, they're content to peck at their feed and stick around the feedhouse. It's the only home they know.

Cage-free means that the chickens are not confined to a tiny cage, but they're still inside a warehouse-type building wing-to-wing with their feathered brethren, barely able to move among their own muck. They have the same little or no access to the outdoors as their free-range brethren.

Organic egg operations feed their chickens organic corn and soy free of antibiotics and pesticides. That's nothing to perform cartwheels about, however, because these chickens can live in the same over-crowded conditions with minimal access to the outdoors.

Pasture-raised eggs are simply the best eggs you can find, and you may need to go to your local farmers market or, at the very least, the health food grocery to find them. But they'll be worth the effort, especially when you see how orange the yolks are. The orange pigment comes from xanthophylls, a class of carotenoids that are healthy for the body.

Eggs got a bad rap for a long time that went like this: *Eggs are high in cholesterol, so they're bad for your heart.* For forty years, this nonsense was repeated. Finally, in 2015, the nation's top nutrition advisory panel, the influential Dietary Guidelines Advisory Committee, said that high-cholesterol foods like eggs do not necessarily affect the level of cholesterol in the blood or increase the risk of heart disease.

Well, hallelujah. Federal health experts have awakened to something I've been saying for fifteen years: eggs are nutritional powerhouses, a nutrient-dense food that packs six grams of protein, a bit of vitamin B_{12}, vitamin E, lutein, riboflavin, folic acid, calcium, zinc, iron, and essential fatty acids into a mere seventy-five calories. Eggs have the highest-quality protein of any food, except for mother's milk.

Notwithstanding the above information about the differing quality of eggs, these incredible edible foods are a major source of allergies. We saw this firsthand after we adopted Samuel when he was six and a half months old. Upon bringing him home, we introduced him to a soft warm egg yolk, as we had done with Joshua. He immediately developed a rash around his mouth. We already knew that he had eczema, as his skin would often become inflamed or irritated.

We immediately stopped giving him egg yolks and waited a year or so until trying again. This time, he did just fine, and we were glad that Samuel grew out of his allergy to eggs, which often happens.

Another important point about eggs: the orange yolk of a pasture-raised egg is really the best part, which makes it so interesting to me that some people throw out the yolk and eat the egg white instead. I know that eating egg whites was popular during the fat-free craze a decade or so ago, as well as in body-building circles, but I believe from a taste and health perspective, the yolk is far superior to the white. This is also true when it comes to allergic potential because the white of the egg contains the more highly allergic proteins.

Perhaps my favorite way to consume pasture-raised eggs is raw in smoothies. While most people are afraid of the germs, I have consumed multiple raw eggs daily for nearly twenty years. I have observed that consuming eggs raw is much less likely to cause allergies.

If you decide to consume raw eggs, make sure to consume organic, pasture-raised eggs. If purchased from a local farm, rinse with warm water and/or hydrogen peroxide and proceed with caution.

3. PEANUTS

Peanuts are probably the best-known allergy among the public because the media will give air time to the local school district banning peanut butter and jelly sandwiches or a major airline refusing a mom's request to advise fellow fliers not to eat nuts because she and her peanut-allergic boy were on the flight. (That actually happened on an American Airlines flight in 2015, and American Airlines canceled the family's seats, which set off a public dispute.) Nearly all airlines have stopped serving small bags of peanuts and replaced them with pretzels or some type of cracker as the drink cart passes through the economy section, while other airlines have discontinued free snacks altogether.

Peanut allergies are real, and it's estimated that approximately one in every 200 persons in the United States has a peanut allergy or at least has to be careful around peanuts. A peanut allergy is different from tree nut allergies, which I'll discuss shortly, because peanuts are technically a legume.

Physical symptoms of an allergic reaction to peanuts range from mild itchiness, swelling, eczema, sneezing, and asthma to more serious manifestations like a drop in blood pressure. In the most severe cases, anaphylaxis—a rapidly progressing, life-threatening episode that includes cardiac arrest—may occur.

I believe a lot of the issues with peanut allergies involve the consumption of peanuts that have been highly hybridized and likely contaminated with the mycotoxin aflatoxin. Produced by the mold *Aspergillus flavus*, aflatoxin is thought to occur in crops that experience extreme heat and drought before harvest, as well as moist, humid storage conditions.

Because peanuts are generally farmed as monocrop agriculture, they are weak and can't resist mold that creates toxins such as aflatoxin. If you have an allergy to peanuts, you should keep your distance.

If you are going to consume peanuts, however, make sure you always purchase organic, which are much less likely to be contaminated. You can also shop for raw varieties of peanuts, including "jungle peanuts" that originate in South America but taste very different from roasted peanuts.

4. TREE NUTS

A tree nut allergy is also one of the most common food allergies in children and adults. Tree nuts such as walnuts, almonds, hazelnuts, cashews, pistachios, and Brazil nuts can cause a severe, potentially fatal, allergic reaction.

According to Food Allergy Research & Education (FARE), an allergy to tree nuts tends to be lifelong. Recent studies have shown that only approximately 9 percent of children with a tree nut allergy will outgrow their allergy. If you have a diagnosed food allergy to tree nuts, they are best avoided. If consuming tree nuts causes minor discomfort including digestive issues, I believe there are ways you can still consume tree nuts and maintain good health by considering the following:

- Consume organic varieties, as some allergic reactions may be due to pesticide and herbicide residue on conventionally raised nuts. If that doesn't make you feel better, then try sprouted nuts and seeds that you have soaked yourself, or you can buy them already soaked and sprouted.

- Soak your nuts, which helps to minimize or eliminate the nutrient inhibitors and toxic substances found in nuts. Soaking may make them more tolerable to those who are sensitive and also increase vitamin B levels and makes the proteins readily available for absorption.

- Another option is to seek out nut butters that are sprouted. Almond, cashew, and mixed nut butters are available in health food stores and may be even easier to digest than sprouted, dehydrated nuts.

- You also might want to think about consuming seeds instead of nuts. I'm a huge believer in the health benefits of sunflower seeds, pumpkin seeds, sesame seeds, flaxseeds, chia seeds, and hemp seeds as they are much less likely to cause allergy, sensitivity, or digestive issues.

I'm seeing a lot of seeds and seed butters in the marketplace such as hemp nut butter, sunflower seed butter, and pumpkin seed butter. If you can kick the nut habit and go with seeds, then you're much more likely to feel a whole lot healthier and better.

5. FISH

Unlike peanut and nut allergies that typically crop up early in infancy and childhood, an allergic reaction to eating fish may not become apparent until adulthood. According to the American College of Allergy, Asthma, & Immunology, as many as 40 percent of people reporting a fish allergy had no problems eating fish until they hit their adult years. That's when they experienced symptoms including:

- tingling or swelling of the lips, tongue, or throat

- abdominal pain

- nausea, vomiting, or diarrhea

- headaches

- asthma

- itching and hives

None of these allergic manifestations are a day at the beach. If any of these symptoms appear regularly after eating a certain type of fish, allergists will recommend that you avoid eating all fish, although through trial-and-error you might be able to safety consume certain fish but not others.

Whether you have a fish allergy or not, I strongly recommend that you avoid fish that troll along the ocean floor or lake bed, where they gobble up gook all day long. I'm talking about species such as sharks and catfish, which are notorious for being "bottom feeders." Sure, they clean up the environment: sharks have a way of vacuuming up the dregs of sea life, and catfish consume fish droppings and any gunk in the water. While it's nice to have these types of fish in our ecosystem, that doesn't mean you should eat them. These fish are more likely to cause health problems because you're eating what *they* ate!

You're going to be so much better off consuming fish with fins and scales caught in the wild. Sockeye salmon, halibut, walleye, and snapper caught in the fullness of nature provide long-chain omega-3 fats, are high in protein, often rich in vitamin D and selenium, and low in toxic metals. Other examples of "healthful" fish include sea bass, cod, sole, and tuna, particularly younger, smaller tuna that are higher in omega-3s and lower in mercury.

What I strongly recommend is that you stay away from farm-raised fish, which is usually sold in stores labeled as "Atlantic salmon" or tilapia. Farm-raised fish aren't raised in the wild and instead pass their days making tight circles in long concrete sloughs or netted pens near coastlines. There's very little room for the fish to move about freely, which doesn't allow the fish the ability to move their muscles naturally.

Farm-raised fish receive hormones to help them grow bigger because of their lack of exercise. They also swim in water that's been treated with chemicals to keep pollution and diseases at bay. These fish aren't eating their natural diet, so their meat doesn't contain nearly as many beneficial omega-3 fatty acids, the prized heart-healthy fats found in many wild fish.

Instead, farm-raised fish are fed pellets made up of genetically modified corn and soy and even poultry litter, and they are administered antibiotics at higher levels than livestock to keep disease at bay in the artificial environment. Synthetic colorants such as canthanxanthin or astaxanthin are added to the feed to give the flesh of farm-raised salmon an appealing orange-hued color because without it, their meat would be a grayish color. How unappetizing would that be?

The smoke-and-mirrors approach is working, however, because in 2011, world farmed-fish production topped beef production. And in 2013, people ate more fish raised on farms than caught in the wild. Nonetheless, you're going to be much better off purchasing and preparing wild-caught fish. My favorites include sockeye salmon from Alaska and deep-water fish such as halibut, which I consume regularly.

Wild-caught tuna is wonderful. Research shows that fattier cuts of tuna contain less mercury than other types because the natural oils contained in fish are detoxifiers of heavy metals. So, when consuming tuna, try to eat the fattier variety, which can be found in health food stores both fresh and canned.

If you have an allergy or sensitivity to fish, it might be because you're eating farm-raised fish. If you know for sure that you're allergic to all fish, including wild-caught, it would be best to avoid consuming them altogether.

6. SHELLFISH

Now here's a class of sea life that in my opinion you should definitely never put on your plate, even though they are among the most popular foods in America and certainly around the world. I'm talking about lobster and shrimp, examples of crustaceans that are served by the millions every day in dishes such as lobster thermidor or shrimp scampi with linguini. That's after an appetizer of fried calamari, which, of course, is another name for squid, also off-limits in my book.

Lobster, shrimp, calamari, crab, crayfish, clams, mussels, oysters, scallops, prawns, and octopus make up a fairly complete listing of the different shellfish commonly eaten in this country. You can add eel and snail to the no-no list, even though they are not shellfish.

I understand the emotional attachment that people have to eating these foods. Some foods—such as lobster—are consumed only on special occasions such as a graduation, an engagement, or a new job. Others enjoy cracking into crab legs and diving into shrimp gumbo at one of those "Bubba" restaurants everyone flocks to on weekends.

That said, I haven't eaten these types of shellfish, at least knowingly, because for over twenty years I've firmly believed that they are unhealthy. Shellfish are problematic for two reasons. Number one, they contain abundant toxins due to their water-bound scavenging habits, and two, shellfish represent a significant risk of allergy to its consumers.

Sure, shellfish clean up the water, but whatever they consume goes straight into their unsophisticated digestive system and, quickly, into their flesh. In fact, scientists gauge the contaminant levels of our oceans, bays, and rivers by measuring the biological toxin levels in the meat of crabs, oysters, clams, and lobsters.

How many stories have we all heard of someone getting sick after eating shellfish? If you often feel queasy after consuming prawns or crayfish, or break out with some sort of skin rash after "enjoying" oysters on the half shell, take that as a warning alarm. Stick to fish with fins and scales, which feed on smaller fish and underwater plant life such as small crustaceans plus algae and seaweed, just as nature intended.

One final thought: you can bet your bottom dollar that if you're allergic to one type of shellfish, then you'll likely be allergic to a wide range of types of shellfish. Science also tells us that if you have a shellfish allergy now, it's likely that you'll never lose this allergy in your lifetime. If you suspect a shellfish allergy, I recommend getting tested and avoid consuming these critters moving forward.

7. SOY

Even though soy is one of the top eight allergy-causing foods, it may surprise you that I don't think soy should be avoided in all cases. There are several foods that are exceptional in the soy category; each are cultured or fermented soy.

Fermentation is key when it comes to soy and allergies. Because proteins cause allergies, anything that breaks down the protein—which fermentation does—usually lowers the likelihood of allergies.

Examples of fermented soy that offer a multitude of health benefits are natto, miso, and unpasteurized soy sauce. Long a popular condiment in Japan, natto has a reputation for being an extremely healthy food with health benefits backed by years of research and studies.

If you've ever wondered why the Japanese population has one of the highest life expectancy rates in the world, then natto has to take partial credit for the way it supports cardiovascular health, a healthy immune system, and digestion. Natto, brimming with beneficial microorganisms, is considered Japan's "miracle food."

The sticking point is taste and aroma. Natto has a stinky smell that can be a stumbling block for American palates. If you're going to give it a try, then natto is best eaten when served over whole-grain brown rice. Actually, make that black rice.

Miso is much better known—and accepted—in this country, where miso soup is often used as a starter in Japanese restaurants. Miso is rich in fiber and high in copper, manganese, vitamin K, and protein. Another Japanese cultured soy product worth mentioning is tempeh, which is similar to a firm vegetarian patty.

Americans are very familiar with soy sauce, which is made from fermented soybeans. When properly prepared and unpasteurized, soy sauce is a healthy, probiotic-rich food. The problem is that commercial soy sauce is manufactured from conventional soybeans *and* pasteurized in addition to containing chemical preservatives.

Soy is one of the more common food allergies, especially among babies and children. Approximately one out of every 250 persons is allergic to soy. Allergic reactions to soy are typically mild, and children generally outgrow the allergy by age three.

The problem for discerning parents is that soy is in *everything*. Well, maybe not everything, but certainly in just about every packaged food sitting on a supermarket shelf. I'm talking baked foods, canned soup, cereals, energy bars, deli meats, vegetable oil, infant formula, and tofu. This means you better be looking on that ingredients label for the words "Contains Soy."

There are many issues with soy beyond the allergies. According to health authors Mannie Barling and Ashley F. Brooks-Simon, food manufacturers add sugar, synthetic sweeteners, genetically modified high-fructose corn sugar, refined salt, artificial flavorings and colors, and monosodium glutamate (MSG) to soy to make it more appetizing. "So soy isn't really soy," wrote Barling and Brooks-Simon. "It is a Frankenfood created for the sole purpose of making a profit from health-conscious people trying to live a healthier life."

Soy comes from soybeans, and I mentioned earlier that 94 percent of the soybean crop in the United States comes genetically modified. This means our soybeans have a gene allowing them to be "Roundup ready," enabling them to be sprayed with pesticides without dying. That pesticide residue becomes part of the food chain.

The additional problem is that soybeans contain phytoestrogens such as isoflavones that mimic the activity of estrogen hormones in the body. Estrogen is normally thought of in terms of female reproduction, but guys need to listen up, too, because estrogens control many aspects of the body for women *and* men, such as metabolism, bone and blood vessel health, skin tone, cholesterol level, fluid balance, and sexual desire.

For me, there are too many issues with soy beyond the allergy situation to regularly consume a food containing soy, unless it is fermented.

8. WHEAT

Wheat allergies, like reactions to soy, are most common in childhood and usually outgrown by the time children reach kindergarten. Wheat allergy is not necessarily the same as gluten sensitivity, but they do produce similar symptoms. I believe that because of the way wheat is hybridized and genetically modified today, most people who suspect a wheat allergy would be better off completely eliminating wheat from their diets, as I talked about in Chapter 6 regarding gluten.

Species related to wheat that are more pure and therefore less hybridized may be easier on the gut; these include einkorn, kamut, and spelt, which may be more tolerable. When in doubt, however, kick all wheat out...of the diet that is. If you insist on consuming wheat and are able to do so without a discernable allergic reaction or sensitivity, I recommend sprouted or whole grain, sourdough whole wheat.

I feel like I covered the issue with the way wheat is raised in this country in Chapter 6, but I want to close with saying that once you improve the health of your gut, I believe you can begin to consume some of the top eight allergens in their best, most digestible form. But for many, a reduction or complete avoidance will be necessary.

TESTING CAN ANSWER KEY QUESTIONS

If you're interested in determining which, if any, foods you're allergic to, I recommend asking your integrative physician to test you using either the ELISA (Enzyme-Linked Immunosorbent Assay) or the ALCAT (Antigen Leukocyte Cellular Antibody Test). Both require a blood draw and can help you determine "hidden" or delayed sensitivities, which provide a level of reactivity that tells you if you have mild or severe allergies to a specific food.

Is there an application to the planet? Sure there is, and it has to do with the way the consumption of the top eight allergenic foods contributes to prescription medication use in affected individuals. The millions who seek relief from their allergies with the use of medications excrete the chemicals they ingest through elimination, which ultimately ends up in our waterways and seeps into our groundwater supply and our soil and, as a result, our crops and even drinking water. Many people suffer from undiagnosed allergies to foods and/or environmental factors and are mistakenly prescribed antibiotics for symptoms that present themselves as bacterial infections.

Avoiding or reducing the consumption of the Allergen Eight and improving our diets by staying away from the foods that cause digestion and immune system problems is a way to indirectly help heal the planet because we'll no longer be excreting as many antibiotics and other medications into our ecosystem.

It's very difficult to determine how the presence of the top eight allergens affects your health, so, when purchasing foods and dietary supplements, I recommend you seek out products that are labeled "Allergen-free" or "Allergen Eight-free."

For more information on foods containing the eight common allergens and their dietary alternatives, visit www.PlanetHealThyself.com.

9

Become an Artisanal Eater

HAVE YOU NOTICED THE LATEST BUZZWORD THESE DAYS—AT LEAST IN food circles?

It's *artisan*.

You can't walk down a supermarket aisle or drive down a main drag without viewing "artisan" on the product packaging or the promotional banners.

Domino's Pizza has a line of rectangular artisan pizzas that feature Alfredo sauce, feta and parmesan-asiago cheese, fresh baby spinach, and chopped onions. Starbucks has their veggie and Monterey Jack artisan breakfast sandwiches. You can find Tostitos Artisan Recipes tortilla chips flavored with grilled red peppers and tomato salsa or roasted garlic and black beans. In the last five years, more than 800 new food products bearing the name "artisan" in the title have emerged out of nowhere.

"The word artisan suggests that the product is less likely to be mass-produced," said Tom Vierhile, innovation insights director at

Datamonitor, a company providing market analysis. "It also suggests that the product may be less processed and perhaps better tasting and maybe even be better for you."

Artisanal foods conjure images of crusty baguettes and stinky European cheese or a craftsman making a high-quality, distinctive product, either by hand or by traditional methods. In some cases and with many common products, that image couldn't be further from the truth. It's easy to be cynical about the flood of artisanal foods because it's obvious that certain corporate marketers are trying to pull the wool over our eyes. They purposely employ the word *artisanal* because they know this carefully researched, focus-grouped, and market-tested adjective works with the buying public and moves product. And because *artisanal* has no legal definition—similar to the words *gourmet* or *natural*—food producers have free rein to do whatever they want.

So how can you, as a consumer, distinguish between a retail gimmick and real artisanal food? The Hartman Group, a food and beverage consulting firm, says that asking three questions will steer you in the right direction. They are:

1. Did a real person craft this food with care?

2. Was this food made by hand, in small batches, or in limited quantities using special ingredients?

3. Does the food product reflect expertise, tradition, passion, and a time-honored process?

It doesn't take a seer to recognize that answering yes to any of these questions would be just about impossible with fast foods, most frozen foods, and nearly all processed foods on supermarket shelves. Even though huge food conglomerates are attempting to co-opt the word *artisan*, I believe we can take back this descriptor, and we do that every time we shop at farmers markets, roadside stands, or the "buy local" sections of health food stores. When we shop for and consume *real* artisanal foods, grown regionally, in a small way we do our part to heal the planet.

Let's start with shopping at farmers markets. When you stroll past the booths and display tables, you can often talk to the farmers who grew the produce, the real-life artisans who baked the irregular-shaped loaves of olive sourdough bread, the local 'preneurs (I think I just made up that word on the spot) who handvrafted the organic mango salsa sold in plastic tubs, or the farmers who grew the imperfectly round heirloom tomatoes.

No matter where you live in the country, you should have a farmers market within reasonable driving distance. Because of rising demand for organic foods—double-digit annual growth has been the norm for more than a decade—farmers markets have been carried along by the same wave of enthusiasm. Farmers markets have more than quadrupled in number since the U.S. Department of Agriculture began keeping records in 1994. Back then, there were 1,755 farmers markets nationwide; by 2014, that number had more than quadrupled to 8,284 and continues to swell.

By definition, a farmers market is a common ground where a handful or several dozen farmers gather on a recurring basis to sell a variety of fresh fruits, vegetables, meats, honey, jams, and other farm products directly to consumers. Farmers markets tend to be concentrated in densely populated areas of the Northeast, Midwest, and West Coast.

One of the pleasant surprises about moving to California during the winter of 2014-15 was discovering San Luis Obispo's Farmers market held every Thursday night in downtown San Luis Obispo. Part street fair, part happening, and all scene, it seemed like the entire community came together to shop for fresh produce, sample delectable cuisine like tri-tip steak and sheep-milk ice cream (yum), check out the craft vendors, foot tap to live music, and watch the kids expend energy in the bounce house or get a hug from Downtown Brown, the farmers market bear mascot. Thousands jam five blocks every Thursday night, rain or shine. The energy and the food were tremendous!

The rapid growth of farmers markets in recent years can be attributed to several factors: a desire to eat local, organic, pesticide-free produce and grass-fed meat, a passion to support local farmers, ranchers, and businesses, an eagerness to build community, and a felt responsibility to know where their food comes from. While some farmers markets have a reputation of catering to certain demographics—empty nesters with disposable income or counterculture free spirits living off the grid—they are becoming more mainstream. Farmers markets appeal to anyone interested in consuming healthier food and leaving a smaller footprint on the planet.

But don't you pay a lot more at farmers markets? Generally speaking, prices are the same or even a bit less than grocery stores because the farmer is selling directly to the consumer with no middlemen involved. I feel you get great value when you buy direct from farmers, the ultimate salt-of-the-earth folks. I've mentioned before how difficult it is grow, cultivate, and bring food to harvest, take it to market, and make enough profit to stay in business, so your purchases can be looked upon as an investment in eco-regeneration.

You can save money if you're flexible, meaning if you're willing to purchase certain seasonal and specialty foods that don't have high demand, such as beets or eggplant. Don't expect to get a bargain, though, during the morning rush between 10 a.m. and noon. You have a better chance of receiving a discount just before closing time because produce is perishable and needs to go. You can also ask if there are any overripe or bruised fruits and veggies available at an advantageous price. Another way to save is to buy in bulk with friends or other families.

Know that with farmers markets, your shopping times are limited. Some markets run only on Saturdays and/or Sundays during the day (usually between 8 a.m. to 2 p.m.); others are open on weekdays in the late afternoon and into the evenings. So you have to build your schedule around the days of operation.

If a spotty timetable doesn't work for you, a great alternative is shopping at roadside stands, which are usually open six or seven days a week. Not only are you buying fresh-from-the-field produce direct from the farmer, but you may get to know him and his family as well. That's what happened to me when we discovered Rutiz Family Farms in Arroyo Grande. I loved the passion for local and organic farming exhibited by owner Jerry Rutiz, who really gets it when it comes to farming fresh produce using regenerative practices, meaning growing healthy plants while building soil fertility.

Jerry shares his farm stand with other vendors' products. You can buy grass-fed beef from rancher Alan Teixeira, ciders and juices from Chadmark Farms in Paso Robles, and artisan breads from Éclair Bakery in Arroyo Grande—the real deal when it comes to artisanal foods. I also took an immediate liking to David's Blue Ribbon Honey, made from European honeybees. Consuming local honey and bee pollen is a great way to stave off allergies.

The Rutiz farm stand is located adjacent to the farm's thirty acres with fifty varieties of harvested crops ranging from sweet corn, tomatoes, artichokes, and cauliflower in summer to cool-weather items like butterleaf lettuce, berries, culinary herbs, and cut flowers. Jerry grows a lot of strawberries, and I loved it during the springtime when they were ripe and luscious. There was a you-pick area, so one morning I rounded up Joshua, Emma, and Alexis and we gathered several quarts of the freshest, reddest, and most succulent strawberries you could sink your teeth into.

What a great learning experience for the kids! Any time you can involve your young children in growing and/or harvesting fruits and vegetables is an awesome way of teaching your children a valuable and tactile understanding of how produce comes from the ground and not a plastic clamshell stacked among dozens of others on an endcap display. My children learned quickly that the best strawberries to pick were the ones without any green or white in the berry and those that they barely tapped and fell out of the plant.

As I watched them survey the strawberry patch like they were on a treasure hunt, I thought about how they have eaten a nearly perfect diet their entire young lives. Perhaps they didn't appreciate the sweet, fresh taste of farm-ripe strawberries like I do. You see, I've eaten junk food in the past (although it's been so long it seems like another life), and I can honestly tell you that these Rutiz strawberries that came off the green plants tasted like candy. Scientists have spent millions of dollars trying to figure out how to create natural strawberry flavoring and artificial strawberry flavoring, but their efforts pale the second you bite into a ripe strawberry picked at the top of the season.

And the eggs…I missed my pasture-raised eggs from the Heal the Planet Farm at the Beyond Organic Ranch, so I shopped for Jerry's pasture-raised beauties…until the day I noticed that he also sold duck and goose eggs.

Goose eggs? That was a new one to me. I mean, I grew up playing baseball, where "goose egg" meant a big, fat zero on the scoreboard. When Jerry showed me his goose eggs, I couldn't get over how massive they were—about four times the size of a regular chicken egg. Harvesting goose eggs wasn't for the faint of heart, either. I learned that you had to sneak up on the goose like a ninja and grab the eggs and get out of there before the goose started biting.

Our sunny-side-up goose eggs were amazing. Someone might say that regular old chicken eggs taste better, but there really wasn't much difference. What my kids really enjoyed was the new experience of breaking open a single egg that filled the entire pan.

ADDITIONAL ARTISANAL AVENUES

I've mentioned farmers markets and roadside stands as options to expand your shopping horizons. I realize that many of you shop at health food stores, just as I have done for years and will continue to do in the future. Modern health food grocery stores are great, and they offer convenient shopping hours and a pleasing environment for their appetizing array of organic fruits and vegetables, grass-fed meats, and wild-caught fish. I love searching and shopping for locally produced artisanal foods at health food stores, which have a knack for displaying products that may not quite be ready for grocery store "prime time."

That's quite alright by me as these retailers are the backbone of the organic-food movement, but wherever you spend your food dollars—at farmers markets, roadside stands, direct from local farmers, or from health food stores—you're casting a vote for organic, non-pesticide, non-GMO, and sustainable foods.

Lastly, I want to put a plug in for specialty markets, especially those that sell the wares of local producers. Independent specialty markets and gourmet grocers are usually the first ones to give new food businesses a try. Specialty stores are where you can find cheese made from sheep's milk, homemade soups, cuts of fresh venison, or certain grass-fed meats like bison and buffalo that you can't find elsewhere. Prices run higher, but so does quality and packaging.

Another way to shop like an artisan is dealing direct with the farmer, like I did when we were living in Florida. I can remember times when I'd drive to a parking lot behind a Palm Beach strip mall to purchase cultured dairy from a local farmer who'd driven into town with picnic coolers topped off with fresh-from-the-pasture raw milk, yogurt, and kefir, eggs, and fresh fruits and veggies. Customers, in turn, brought their own coolers and cash.

I was recently able to make a connection with a local couple, Greg and Lindy, with access to a couple of cows. Not only that, but Greg was a fisherman and recently sent me a text message that he'd caught wild king salmon off of California's central coast and asked if I wanted to try some. Boy did I! There's nothing quite like a dinner of fresh-caught wild salmon over black rice and complemented with organic corn and peas.

The fisherman's wife, Lindy, and I got to talking about raw milk, and the next thing I knew I was making arrangements to buy raw milk from her. We miss our cows and dairy operation back in Missouri, but it wasn't practical to ship raw milk across the country, so supporting a local artisan who could supply us with fresh raw milk was a bonus.

You become a food artisan yourself when you seek out small, independent dairymen, farmers, and ranchers. You have to be willing to strike up conversations with people you don't know at roadside stands and farmers markets, which can be difficult, but once you do, you plug into a whole new way of living. By introducing yourself in a friendly manner and engaging in give-and-take conversation, you build a network and learn things that you never thought you would.

When locals learned that we had recently moved to Arroyo Grande, they asked us if we had visited nearby attractions. I'd heard of Hearst Castle north of San Luis Obispo off Highway 1, so taking the family there was fun. But I hadn't heard of Guadalupe-Nipomo Dunes, the largest intact coastal dune system on Earth. Undulating for eighteen miles along the Central California shore, Nipomo Dunes stretches from Pismo Beach to Point Sal. A steady wind sweeps over the area, sculpting the sand into towering peaks that stretch five hundred feet heavenward.

I learned a bit of trivia during our visit: the 1923 silent film *The Ten Commandments* was filmed there by Cecil B. DeMille and his crew, and archeologists and tourists are *still* finding artifacts and parts of the movie set more than ninety years later. (DeMille remade *The Ten Commandments* in 1956 with Charlton Heston as Moses and a cast of thousands.) We didn't find any plaster sphinxes, but it was a great family outing.

One area close to our new home in California that I wanted to show the kids was Salinas, a fertile valley south of San Jose and a bit east of Monterey. Along Highway 101, there were green fields of iceberg, green leaf, and red leaf lettuce, endive, kale, and parsley. Salinas wasn't called the "Salad Bowl of America" for nothing.

Sure, it was mostly conventional, monocrop agriculture, but it was still impressive nonetheless to speed past mile-long rows of various greens. Several farms happened to be fertilizing that day, so when the sulfur-like smell invaded our car filled with two adults and six children, a blame game ensued among the kids, who accused each other of having let one go.

ACTING ARTISANAL

When you step away from the conventional food shopping matrix, you have the opportunity to buy, prepare, and consume food that's artisanal in the original sense of the word. That's why my encouragement to you is to become artisanal in your outlook, someone who fully appreciates food for everything it represents as a profound understanding of the craft of making meals. Even if you don't cook much, food artisans are environmentally conscious and don't waste anything.

Hundreds or even thousands of years ago, food artisans of that day invented fermentation to preserve juice, milk, bread, and meat for a longer period of time. These food artisans understood and respected the foods they worked with, knew what good food should taste like, and mastered processes such as bread-making, cheese-making, micro-brewed beers, charcuterie, drying meats, and making sushi, to list a few examples. They had a deep love for their craft, for the food they ate, and for those who enjoyed their foods.

You can, too. I think being an artisan is a great way to go through life and can expand your horizons. I've lived a short time in several places throughout my forty years of life. I've also visited hundreds of small towns, medium-sized cities, and major metropolises in the continental U.S., but I've never been in a place like San Luis Obispo County where people I met generally made statements like, *I've been here ten years, and it's paradise* or *I would never live anywhere else...we love it here.*

I could see what they were talking about just from our short time here in Arroyo Grande. Our front yard and backyard was home to grapevines, a guava tree, a lime tree, blueberry bushes, a small straw-berry patch, and a prolific lemon tree. I have consumed the juice of two or three lemons a day in my various super drinks and then "recycled" the spices by tossing the used-up ginger, turmeric, clove, and cinnamon bark as mulch in the flower beds.

I got into the habit of picking my lemons in bare feet because years ago I learned about a concept called *earthing*, also known as *grounding*. Walking on the grass each day not only gave me a connection to the earth but also put me in touch with beneficial microorganisms found in grass and dirt. Plus it felt darn good to feel the earth squish between my toes with each step.

This was the first time I'd ever lived in a home with "edible landscaping" as opposed to our years in South Florida suburbia where everything grown was ornamental—from Queen palm trees to azalea shrubs to dragon's breath plants.

As an East Coaster all my life, I had formed opinions about people on the Left Coast. California had a reputation as the land of fruits and nuts, populated with high-stress people who were stuck in traffic all the time. And all they ate was Mexican food and In-and-Out Burgers.

After spending a year in Central California, though, I was genuinely impressed with the friendliness of the locals and how they weren't into fast food. In fact, it was just the opposite. Many people I met were into something called the "slow food" movement, which was a bit ironic because we were living near SLO—pronounced *slow* by San Luis Obispo locals. At any rate, slow food is a way of saying no to the rise of fast food and a fast life. Slow food means living in an unhurried manner and taking time to enjoy life's simple pleasures.

Leaving the hustle and bustle of South Florida for a Missouri farmstead and then taking a detour to Central California provided a way for my family and me to step back and embrace a slower pace. We aren't alone. There's actually an international movement called Slow Food that was organized thirty years ago by an Italian journalist, Carlo Petrini, in response to the opening of a McDonald's in the shadow of Rome's Spanish Steps. Talk about a *mama mia* for Petrini, who despised the notion of junk food being sold near such a revered landmark. He promoted the idea of Slow Food as way to preserve traditional and regional cuisine while encouraging sustainable farming and meat-raising that benefited the local ecosystem.

Over two decades, the Slow Food movement has expanded globally to over 100,000 members in 150 countries with the idea of fighting back against the globalization of agriculture products by promoting local small farms. A few years ago, I attended a chapter meeting of Slow Food in South Florida and left favorably impressed with what they were trying to do.

I love how the Slow Food movement is a counterweight to the busyness of life that constantly tugs at our ankles. Taking time to think through what we should eat, how we should shop, and what kind of pleasures are important to us are steps we can take to preserve biodiversity and have an artisanal mindset.

Eat local and eat slow.

Sounds like a great way to heal our bodies and our planet.

For more information on eating as an artisan, including links to farmers market directories and wonderful eco-friendly farms in the U.S., visit www.PlanetHealThyself.com.

10

Heal the Planet: Living the Eco-Regenerative Lifestyle

YOU MAY HAVE NOTICED A WORD IN THE CHAPTER TITLE THAT'S PROBA-
bly new to you: *eco-regenerative.*

This coined word is shorthand for "regeneration of our living ecology." There are other words or phrases used to describe how we can act favorably to the environment—such as "going green" or "living sustainably"—but at the end of the day, it's all about the little steps we can all take to contribute to the health of the planet.

One big step that I'm taking both personally and professionally to be more eco-regenerative is to take part in an initiative to lighten the burden of consumer packaging on the planet. You see, before I purchased Missouri farmland, I lived in South Florida, where I was founder and CEO of a health and nutrition company that grew big enough to produce millions of bottles of nutritional supplements each year. I'm talking about plastic and glass bottles with a plastic lid filled with tablets, capsules, and powders…just like the thousands of other products that fill aisles in grocery stores, big-box outlets, health food stores, supplement shops, and pharmacies everywhere.

The company I started was acquired in 2009, and I decided to become an organic farmer. In 2015, I started a new company called Get Real Nutrition, and this time, I'm taking the proverbial bull by the horns when it comes to being an eco-regenerative, socially responsible, consumer-packaged goods company.

As my team and I discussed packaging, I thought, *It's déjà vu all over again—all those plastic bottles and plastic lids made from petrochemicals headed for the landfill or at best the recycling bin. Is there something we can do to reduce or even reverse our carbon footprint?*

Everyone knows that materials ending up in landfills take years and years to break down and create methane gases that cause problems as well. But was there a way we could be part of the solution instead of part of the problem?

I thought back to my Grandpa Jerry, who turned his Long Island backyard into a vegetable garden and composting pit that I experienced nearly every summer as a child. Papa Jerry laid down strips of newspaper when planting a new row of vegetables and ripped cardboard into smaller pieces and tossed it into his beloved compost pile, along with sections of the *New York Times*. Adding newspaper and paper products is a common practice for composters because paper is a biodegradable product of trees, but the carbon-based black ink that many newspapers use isn't the most environmentally friendly.

The other issue is that when you take packaged material that *is* compostable but toss it into the kitchen trash—where it eventually makes its way to a landfill—that packaged material will break down, but it won't be truly composted. Soil-producing composting is the gold standard when it comes to regeneration because the practice creates much-needed topsoil that can heal the planet.

In the last few years, when I've shopped at natural food grocery stores, I've seen multicolored bins marked "Trash" and "Recycling," but recently I've noticed green bins marked "Composting," especially near the deli sections and cafes. The composting bin is for items like apple cores, banana skins, watermelon rinds, salad leaves, bread scraps, and cardboard—I'm barely scratching the surface.

Which got me thinking…what if the packaging material from foods and supplements could go into the composting bin instead of the blue recycling container? Or, as I asked my team, was it possible to produce packaging material that was completely renewable and environmentally friendly, even made without the black and ultraviolet glossy color inks that are problematic?

I knew there were inks made of soybean- and plant-based components that could be broken down in a composting environment. We decided that utilizing those environmentally friendly elements would produce packaging that would be made up of completely compostable and/or purposed recyclable material.

We also decided to look at everything else we were doing in an environmental light. In fact, if you're holding a physical copy of *Planet Heal Thyself* in your hands, then you're reading a book made up of compostable materials. We also launched a periodical called *Get Real Magazine* that's comprised of compostable paper as well.

We see this, corporately speaking, as our way to bring an eco-regenerative ethos to our brand. If you happen to purchase our products, I want to share some ideas that we want to encourage you to do as your part to heal the planet. When it comes to our products' outer cartons, *Get Real Magazine,* our company literature, product displays, and as mentioned, this book (if you're done reading it and don't have anyone to pass it along to, that is), we recommend the following:

1. Compost it yourself. I described composting in Chapter 3 in great detail, which could be more accurately called vermicomposting because of the way worms—*vermi* is Latin for worm—break down the organic material.

2. Take the packaging materials to a local farm. Farmers are always looking for ways to fertilize and build their soil. Nearly all farms, especially smaller ones, have soil-building composting piles in place. If convenient, you can contribute not only your packaging materials but also your organic food waste. Believe me, your local farmer would love you!

3. Bring the packaging materials to a local drop-off center. Many progressive health food stores and grocery stores have industrial composting systems where you can drop off your compostable materials to be composted.

4. We are working on a way to pick up—at least in Southern Missouri—compostable materials. Then we will transport them to our soil-building system at the Heal the Planet Farm.

When thinking about a completely closed loop system of preservation and regeneration, I had a phrase come to me: "Today's packaging is tomorrow's nutrition."

When you purchase nutritional supplements, foods, or beverages that come packaged in compostable materials, you're essentially saying with your purchase is that today's packaging becomes tomorrow's nutrition because when you compost packaging material, it creates soil that can be used to grow food and provide nutrients for you or someone else.

I'd say that's a pretty cool way to heal the planet.

POST-CONSUMER RECYCLING

In my mind as a business owner and entrepreneur (or what I prefer to call myself, a missionpreneur), the ultimate standard in packaging is something called "post-consumer recycled material," which means a company produces their packaging from materials that have already been recycled. There's something beautiful for the planet when one material is reused to produce something different, like turning old printing paper into paperboard, for example.

You can also turn plastic grocery bags, bread bags, case over-wrap, dry cleaning bags, newspaper sleeves, ice bags, Ziploc and other re-sealable bags, produce bags, and bubble wrap into eco-friendly composite decking made from a blend of 95 percent recycled wood and plastic. That's what a progressive company called Trex Recycling is doing—recycling plastic material into decking material for backyards and playgrounds.

Trex has partnered with grocery retailers like Albertsons, A&P, Safeway, Sprouts Farmers market, Winn-Dixie, and Whole Foods as places where consumers can bring their plastic bags and wrappings that will be turned into composite decking. In other words, today's packaging can become tomorrow's playground. What a neat way to lighten the load that today's consumption of resources has on the planet.

Trex does not accept plastic bottles because the cost to ship them to their recycling facility is prohibitive, but there are plenty of other options to recycle plastic bottles. Most plastic bottles are tossed into a blue recycling bin that goes out to the curb, where they're picked up and taken to a recycling center. The trash gets dumped onto a conveyor belt, and the plastic bottles get separated from glass and paper by machines and human "pickers." The bottles are then crushed into a bale, wrapped up, stacked on wooden pallets, and shipped off to various after-market manufacturers that turn plastic bottles into stain-resistant carpet, fleece clothing, or into plastic bottles again.

It's really amazing how much bottled water we drink each year—around 50 billion disposable bottles worth. We used to drink significantly more soft drinks, but according to the International Bottled Water Association, bottled water is expected to overtake soft drinks as the number-one packaged beverage sold in the U.S. in 2016. While it's great to see Americans develop a thirst for water over unhealthy soft drinks comprised of sugar, high fructose corn syrup, and artificial sweeteners, drinking water from plastic bottles is not the best way to heal the planet.

Sure, the convenience and portability of bottled water can't be beat, but if you're drinking bottled water at home or grabbing a bottle when you jump in the car to do errands, you're contributing to a huge landfill problem. The average American drinks 167 disposable water bottles each year but only recycles 38 of them, which means a recycling rate of 23 percent.

Any sort of plastic container takes years or decades to break down when it reaches a landfill. Even glass, which comes from earth materials, is very difficult to break down. There are challenges finding the right materials—ones that can be easily recycled—in packaging for the commercial market.

And then I heard about a community of sustainable leaders who came together to drive change in the natural products industry—in the area of packaging. As this small group talked about working together to create positive change, they decided to name their budding organization One Step Closer to an Organic and Sustainable Community, or OSC[2].

This consortium is an amalgamation of progressive and forward-thinking organic companies that span food, beverage, skin care, and dietary supplement categories. Companies such as Alter Eco,

Guayaki Organic Yerba Mate, Happy Baby, 18 Rabbits, and Mary's Gone Crackers have banded together to find compostable and sustainable packaging solutions. We—referring to Get Real Nutrition—were invited to join this organization, and we readily said yes. We're sitting next to CEOs of brands such as Numi Organic Tea and Nutiva—products that my family personally enjoys—and working together on ways to not only create sustainable and regenerative packaging solutions for our companies but also to lead the way for others.

I urge you to seek out and support the brands that are part of OSC² the next time you're in a health food store or natural grocers. You can find out more about OSC² at osc2.org.

We're excited to discover ways to decrease and even reverse our carbon footprint and produce products that have compostable and recyclable materials—and think outside the box when it comes to the way we package our products.

One way we've decided to accomplish this is to make our Get Real Nutrition supplements the first encapsulated dietary supplement brand packaged without bottles. Instead, we will package our organic, encapsulated products into a pouch dropped into a rectangular cardboard box, which will greatly reduce the amount of plastic that ends up in landfills. In fact, our 100 percent recyclable packaging contains nearly 90 percent less petro-plastic resin than plastic bottles and weighs significantly less than glass bottles, which reduces the fossil fuels used to distribute the products.

We are also partnering with Trex Recycling so that our packaging today can perhaps become tomorrow's playgrounds.

PACKAGING AND TRANSPORTATION

Now I'd like to bring in our environmental specialist, Jason Dewberry, Chief Marketing Officer of Get Real Nutrition. Jason, who's worked closely with me for fifteen years, will answer some questions about how individuals' purchasing habits and where they choose to spend their money can have a lasting impact on the environment. I've charged Jason with the assignment of coming up with environmentally friendly/eco-regenerative packaging for Get Real Nutrition.

So Jason, what kind of impact are we having today as a nation that largely subsists on food and products packaged in petroleum-based packaging? In other words, how big is the issue?

Jason Dewberry: Let me answer your question by saying that the Industrial Revolution of the 18th and 19th centuries did create a lot of advancements in society at an economic level, but that we are now paying the price with our health. But it's not just our health; it's the health of our planet.

At one time, we were consuming whole, unrefined, un-synthesized, and natural foods that were grown in our own communities and transported by animals within walking proximity to the village. Today, we can see how the requirements to package these foods and bring them to market has left a huge toll on the environment.

You have factories cranking out all this carbon monoxide into the atmosphere to produce the food, and then when the food items come off of the assembly line in plastic and cardboard containment units, they have to be transported and shipped to stores, which leaves another carbon footprint. But what's interesting to me is the trend toward single-unit, single-person, single-meal packaging like you get with a Lunchable or some type of snack-like packaging. Our kids are growing up thinking that this "one-off" food is very normal to eat, which is a drastic departure from the way we grew up.

And about the way our foods get to market...for a long time in our history, all of our foods got to market in a wagon, pulled by a horse. Now we are dependent on 18-wheelers and tractor-trailers, coal-burning trains, coal-burning ships, and wide-body jet aircraft—all of which run on fossil fuels. And we're just as dependent on the oil to produce the plastic containers, bottles, clamshells, bags, and pouches, which is an interesting parallel.

So when we talk about regeneration in body, mind, and planet, it isn't just a fancy phrase or clever hook that a marketer is going to use to get somebody's attention. We have to come up with a solution that's going to impact the soil, our bodies, as well as the planet.

Jordan: Talk about the use of petroleum-based packaging. The truth is, when we go to a supermarket or a health foods store, even the bulk produce we buy goes in a plastic bag prior to checkout. There has to be tons of those plastic bags as well as plastic bottles clogging up landfills. What problems does this cause?

Jason: Even with all the technology around us, it's like we're dying of thirst in a sea of water. It's like we have the answers all around us, but we can't see them. They're hidden in plain sight.

If you just carve out one tiny piece of our food chain in the industrial food complex and just look at water bottles, for example, you realize that it's a staggering amount. Think of the billions of bottles out there not only for the water industry but for the juice industry, the soda industry, or any ready-to-drink beverage that lines the shelves of conventional grocery stores. It's overwhelming, and the true definition of unsustainable.

The reason I say unsustainable is simply because right now, 99 percent of the plastics made globally are dependent upon oil for their source. Oil is a finite resource, which is why I say utilizing petroleum-based plastics is unsustainable, especially at the rate we're consuming them today.

In terms of minimizing the amount of plastic and packaging we're dependent on, we have to make a tangible impact generationally. That's something that we're passionate about doing at Get Real Nutrition.

Sure, whatever we can accomplish in recyclable and compostable packaging would be like picking up a few grains of sand on a beach, but what we are trying to do is prove a concept and show that the technology is there to be better, to do better.

I mean, take the simple notion about filling up bottles. In the nutritional supplement industry, the current model today is utilizing plastic, petroleum-based bottles that often times get filled to just one-third capacity but rarely much more than 65-70 percent and stuffed with GM bleached cotton. The reason the bottle has to be so big is for "shelf impact," but at the end of the day, we have billions of these oversized bottles getting thrown away and ending up in landfills.

Are some of the bottles diverted to recycling? I suppose so, but a lot of these plastic bottles are made with resins that make them unsuitable for the recycling industry. So Jordan, when you and I started talking about launching a new brand, we discussed the available packaging that's out there and how some companies "greenwash"—claiming they are environmentally friendly when they aren't. We definitely wanted to do more, and the concept that we keyed in on was the tagline, "Thinking outside the bottle."

We're swimming against the current stream in our industry by being the first brand in our class to deliver our dietary supplements outside the bottle. We are reducing the amount of petroleum-based resin by a factor of 90 percent. Ours is a holistic solution that not only impacts our business model but also gives us a consumer education opportunity. We are also challenging our industry to do better than what they've been doing for the last twenty or thirty years. A lot of the bigger companies and brands haven't invested in this new biodegradable, renewable, compostable, 100 percent recyclable packaging technology that we've found.

Jordan: Why don't you tell everyone the steps we've come up with to help consumers lighten the load on the planet.

Jason: Glad to do it, and there are three simple recommendations:

1. When you're shopping, bring your own bag.

Municipalities around the country are banning plastic bags, which create huge litter problems as well. Have you seen all the plastic bags blown by the wind into shrubs and trees? Looks trashy, too.

2. Educate yourself on what is truly recyclable and then buy those products.

Look for the green logos on the packaging.

3. Invest in and/or buy products in compostable packaging.

I know Jordan has already explained his compostable packaging ideas. If you don't compost yourself, make sure to put your compostable materials into industrial composting receptacles found at most health food stores and groceries. Or you can go to a local farm such as the Heal the Planet Farm that will take today's packaging and turn it into tomorrow's nutrients.

Jordan: Why do you think the marketplace has been slow to adopt these solutions?

Jason: Because consumers aren't asking for it, not demanding it enough. By way of illustration, Frito-Lay produces SunChips, a brand of snack chips. Frito-Lay pioneered a 100 percent compostable bag for their SunChips but ended up scrapping it because focus groups and too many consumers complained because it was a different kind of plastic and a different kind of bag that was a little bit more rigid and crinkly—and too loud. The noise upon opening turned out to be an issue for many customers.

Talk about how no good deed goes unpunished. So Frito-Lay moved away from the 100 percent compostable bags to something like 30 percent compostable bags, which means opportunity lost. It's a combination of big businesses not really investing all the way in more sustainable packing, but even more the consumer mindset needs to shift away from its *I'm not used to something new* mentality.

We've all heard the phrase, "Vote with your dollar." From my standpoint, I would ask people to go a little bit further and do the research and support the brands investing in sustainable or, better yet, eco-regenerative packaging technologies.

Your voice can also be heard, like those who complained about noisy SunChips. Every consumer-packaged good has a throwaway phrase on the back of their package: *For your comments and feedback, we would love to hear from you.*

You can send your feedback via email or by calling a toll-free number. If you like what they're doing, tell them. If you think they could do better, tell them!

Jordan: Those are great ideas. I guess the bottom line here is that when companies are making positive efforts, we need to let them know.

We also live in a society where consumer-goods packaging is critical. Just to give you an example, I recently made two smoothies in the morning, which is my habit because we're a family of eight. In one of the smoothies, I used fresh-pressed apple juice that I got from a health foods store that came in a plastic container. I used bananas where the only unsustainable thing on the fruit was the sticker on the peel, so that was pretty good. I used kale and spinach, and both of those came in plastic clamshell-type containers. They're certainly healthy and fresh, but they still came in plastic containers.

I added frozen açai puree that came in a plastic pouch with an outer plastic package, and then I had frozen organic blueberries that came in a little plastic bag. So my smoothie that was comprised entirely of single-ingredient fresh and frozen foods still came in lots of packaging.

The point is we're going to consume lots of products and packaging, even if we consume fresh, organic, and whole single-ingredient foods. So when it comes to influencing what happens in the world today, we should support companies that produce packaging that avoids going in the landfill through strategic recycling plans and compostable packaging.

Jason was absolutely right about voting with your dollar for companies that use eco-regenerative packaging and do things well for our bodies and the planet.

HEALING THE PLANET THE PERMACULTURE WAY

I described in the Introduction of *Planet Heal Thyself* how I became interested in permaculture, a system of living in such a way that you leave the planet in better condition than you found it. I also introduced Bill Wilson, the founder of Midwest Permaculture, who was partially responsible for raising my consciousness about the way we farm in this country and why we need to protect and *build* topsoil—before it's too late.

Bill and I have gotten to know each other pretty well in the last year or so, and he's been advising me on how to apply the concepts of permaculture to our organic ranching and farming efforts in Southern Missouri. As I got to know Bill and his wife, Becky, we kicked around several ideas, including one I had about carving out 320 acres (out of nearly 4,000 total acres) to become the Heal the Planet Farm. More ideas poured forth, including building a "demonstration farm" that could show the world what can be done to heal the land and leave it in a far better condition than how we found it.

Throughout the rest of this chapter, I'll be sharing Bill's permaculture vision for the Heal the Planet Farm using his PowerPoint presentation on permaculture that he presents whenever he travels around the country speaking on this topic. But first I want you to hear from him how he became interested in permaculture.

Bill Wilson: I'm not as young as I used to be, but when I was around twenty-two years old, I realized that how we live on the planet makes a huge difference in the quality of life for future generations. I felt a sense of responsibility to do something, but I didn't know what to do or how to go about it.

At the same time, I woke up to the idea that food is your best medicine, which makes food and our ability to continue to *grow* food really important. The idea of living sustainably on the land and caring for nature resonated with me. I thought there were ways we could live on the planet without going backward because no one wants to live in a cave or a teepee. So the question became: how can we as a society move forward and have abundance while leaving the planet in a better condition than when we arrived?

Back in the late 1970s, I heard about a small community in Illinois that was sustainably oriented—early adopters, if you will. Stelle, located seventy-five miles south of Chicago, was an unincorporated township of just one hundred residents. What was unique about Stelle—and still is today—was that many residents were interested in gardening, solar energy, wind power, and community living long before they became part of the national conversation.

I drove to Stelle in 1978 to check it out, and I'm still here nearly forty years later. There's no doubt that being part of the Stelle community has exposed me to living more consciously and more sustainably than the average American. We use about one-third less energy, grow as much of our food as we can, and buy as much as we can from local farmers and ranchers. We're not 100 percent self-sustainable, far from it really, but we're certainly moving in the right direction. We have a garden co-op, a chicken co-op, and even a tool co-op.

For years, I told Becky that I ached for there to be a way that we as humans could live on the planet and leave it in a better condition when we left. Becky felt the same way, so we took steps to turn this deep interest in permaculture into a vocation. After taking the necessary courses from permaculture trainers, it became crystal clear that we as the human family could live abundantly well with a high quality of life and still live sustainably.

Somehow I needed to make permaculture my life's work, and with Becky on board, we co-founded Midwest Permaculture in 2007. We put on seminars and offer week-long courses providing students a Permaculture Design Certificate (PDC). We've grown every single year and have over 1,000 graduates.

Often times when I introduce people to permaculture, they say to me, "Oh, my gosh! I've thought about that and believed that way all my life. You mean there's a word for that?"

That's our goal—to make permaculture a household word. Our objective is to look at the world through a clear lens and make decisions based on the greatest care for others and the planet.

Permaculture is best exemplified when there is a convergence of common sense, indigenous wisdom, and appropriate technology. It's about being intelligent, creative human beings, assessing the situation, and making choices that advance the human experience on this planet while caring for creation at the same time. Our objective is to design livable systems for people that support and mimic nature's own ability to create abundance.

Jordan: That's a great introduction. Now I want you to share some excerpts from your permaculture presentation and introduce the Heal the Planet Farm:

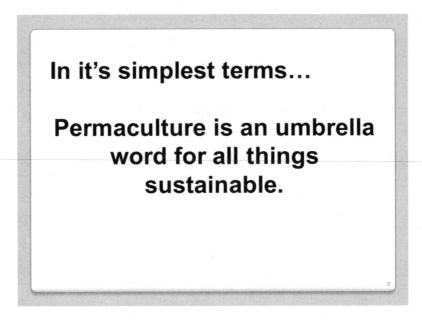

In it's simplest terms…

Permaculture is an umbrella word for all things sustainable.

Bill: Glad to do it. We often have a booth at various state fairs, and I'll have a hundred people come up to me in a day and ask, "What's permaculture?"

The simplest answer is that permaculture is an umbrella word for all things sustainable. Whether we're talking about renewable energy, water harvesting, energy-efficient homes, growing food, or raising livestock, it all falls under the umbrella of permanent culture.

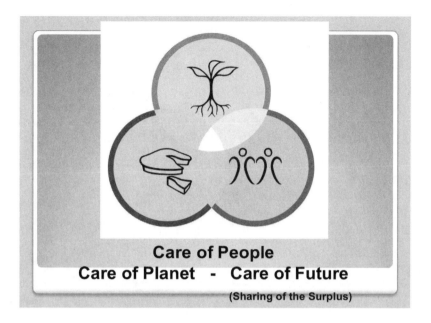

Care of People
Care of Planet - Care of Future
(Sharing of the Surplus)

Permaculture is a design science that's practical, realistic, and works with nature to design systems that are long term and sustainable. Our intention is to care for creation—the planet, the land, and the people for future generations.

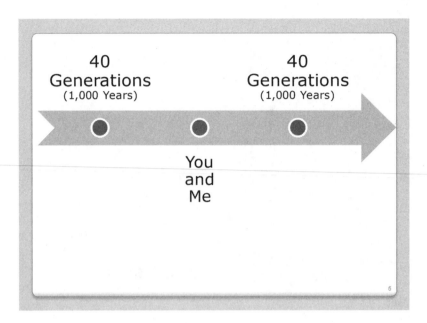

We tend to think of ourselves as being pretty important in this present day and age. That's true to a certain extent, but if you look at a spectrum of 2,000 years, you can see that the span of our lifetimes is fairly insignificant. Yet when we put everyone together, you can see that we all have a huge impact positively or negatively.

Permaculture is inviting us to answer the question, "How can we live responsibly?" Permaculture is thinking about the future of the planet rather than just our own lifetime.

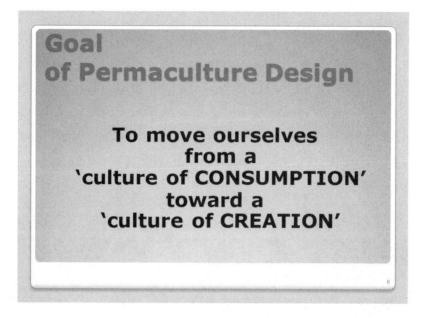

It's only been in the last one hundred years that we've become a consumptive culture. Before then, by and large, we were farmers, we were craftsmen, and we were skilled individuals providing something for our communities. We created things. Now we consume them.

Not only do we consume, but when we're done, we throw it away, which means we have a trash problem. It's said that 90 percent of everything manufactured this year will be in the trash next year.

Permaculture is a response to overconsumption. If all we do is consume and consume, we're destroying the planet for future generations. That's irresponsible and certainly not sustainable.

Jordan: It's becoming clearer that we've become a nation of mass consumers, but that's created a major set of issues.

Even if we didn't change our consumption model, the fact that we're eating so much food and not utilizing our natural resources properly is problematic. If we were to take all the consumer waste products from the foods we eat and utilize permaculture principles, we could turn things around quickly.

It's amazing how we have completely handicapped ourselves. In the Introduction, I talked about how the soil in Illinois is the envy the world, but 95 percent of everything big eaten in Illinois comes from out of state! Midwest Permaculture is trying to get its message out to one person, one backyard, and one community at a time.

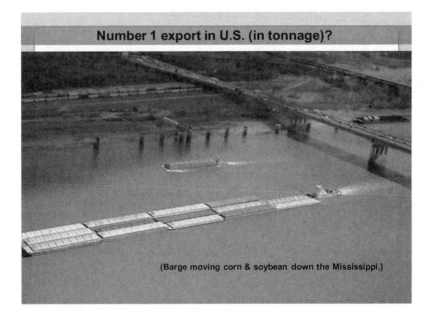

Number 1 export in U.S. (in tonnage)?

(Barge moving corn & soybean down the Mississippi.)

Bill: When I talk about consumption, this is mindboggling. If you look at that barge moving down the Mississippi River and ask the question *What's the number-one export in the U.S.?* most people would answer "corn."

If you remember from Jordan's Introduction, the number-one export is actually topsoil. This picture is evidence that they don't call the Mississippi River the "Big Muddy" for nothing. We lose an incredible amount of topsoil every year—1.9 billion tons. That would fill enough rail cars to wrap around the globe seven times.

There's also wind erosion that's scraped off layers of topsoil. The way we farm on a big scale does a number on soil fertility as well. There's no way to practice annual tillage without damaging or losing the soil.

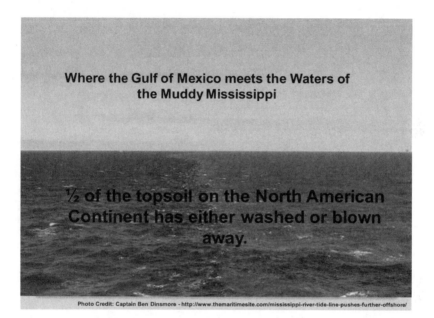

Where the Gulf of Mexico meets the Waters of the Muddy Mississippi

½ of the topsoil on the North American Continent has either washed or blown away.

Photo Credit: Captain Ben Dinsmore - http://www.themaritimesite.com/mississippi-river-tide-line-pushes-further-offshore/

This illustration shows the definitive line where the muddy Mississippi connects with the fresh clear waters of the Gulf of Mexico. Not only are we losing so much topsoil, but we're also losing a lot of nitrogen fertilizer. About one-third of all nitrogen fertilizer ends up in the water table and in our rivers in the central part of the United States.

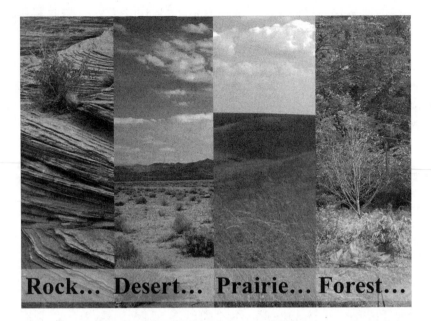

Rock... Desert... Prairie... Forest...

This gives a simple, practical example of what a permaculture design on the landscape might look like.

So, imagine that you and I are standing on a rock, and as far as the eye can see, there's rock everywhere. But we have a half a bushel of garden seeds, so we're going to take the garden seeds, throw them out on the rock, and stand here for a growing season.

The sun comes up every day, and once in a while it rains. But what's our yield? What can we expect to harvest by throwing seed out onto a stone? Pretty much nothing.

Now put 2-3 feet of topsoil on those rocks and throw the exact same seeds out there...and what's your yield? Most likely, a lot. That is why topsoil is so important.

But now let's suppose it's not we who are standing on this rock with three feet of soil on top. Let's pretend our parents are standing on this rock twenty, thirty, or forty years ago, and they throw some seeds out because they want to eat this year, but they also plant walnut, oak, chestnut, and hickory trees. These nut trees, when they finally mature, produce a nut crop so great that you can barely walk underneath the tree's canopy because there are so many nuts on the ground.

And in front of those nut trees, our parents put in a standard variety of fruit trees—massive cherry, apple, and plum trees. And berry bushes, like gooseberries and currents. And in front of the berries, they put in asparagus and rhubarb.

In other words, they planted forty or fifty different crops that are perennial in nature, and they don't have to do anything to them because those plants continue to produce crops year after year. Sure, they had to wait four or five years for the trees and shrubs to gain some maturity, but within a generation their yields become massive, much more there than they could ever possibly eat in a single growing season.

It's not just the food, though, that they've grown. The trees provide wood. They need fuel, and they need to build a house. They need shade, they need protection from the wind, and it's there.

This is what a permaculture design is. And how much work did we do over the last twenty-five years to develop that? We didn't do squat. It was our parents who had the foresight to plant years ago. That's the abundance of nature that we're talking about.

If we work with nature to design systems that will be abundant over time, we do less and less work as we produce more and more yield. That's what we're after.

So take another look at this illustration. You see pictures of rock, desert, prairie, and forest. Here's another example of this: Imagine you and your family are out on a cruise or a ship somewhere. The ship goes down, and everybody perishes but you and the family. You end up on a deserted island, and that's where you're going to spend the rest of your lives. Do we want that island to be rock, sand, or desert? Or prairie? Or would you like it to be a forest?

Isn't it clear to you that the forest environment is where abundance shows up for the human species? It's really the trees in the forest that have made it possible for the human species to live abundantly well on this planet.

Without forests, the landscape gets dryer and dryer and dryer. You have less and less rain, you have less water soaking into the soil, and so to reverse that—to recharge the environment—you have to heal the landscape, and that takes water.

The first step in permaculture is to hold water on the landscape… as high up as possible.

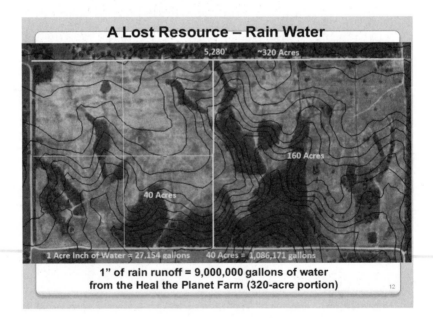

A Lost Resource – Rain Water

5,280'   ~320 Acres

160 Acres

40 Acres

1 Acre Inch of Water = 27,154 gallons   40 Acres = 1,086,171 gallons

1" of rain runoff = 9,000,000 gallons of water
from the Heal the Planet Farm (320-acre portion)

Jordan: Bill, let me jump in here with the next illustration. I've heard you say in the past that one of the keys to permaculture is to make sure that we have an environment of retaining water, which absolutely blew me away when I started doing the math on how much water we lose whenever there's a big rain.

These next few illustrations lay out how Midwest Permaculture is working with the Heal the Planet Farm to design maximum water holding capacity, optimal soil fertility, and the ability for us to convert the elements of nature into nutrition.

Can you explain to us how much water comes from an inch of rain, how much the land can hold, and the steps that the Heal the Planet Farm is taking to address this?

Bill: When you invited me to consider working with you, I did some research and pulled up a map of your land. With the software programs I have, I can lay topographical lines on the maps and see instantly that you have a 100-foot drop from the top of your property to the bottom. That's quite a bit of slope.

I thought to myself, *Boy, I sure hope those pastures are really solid and strong because when they get a good rain, they're losing a lot of water moving off that landscape.* And then I found out from you that your pastures are not as strong as you would like.

You asked how much water there is in an inch of rain. It's understood that if an inch of rain falls on an acre-sized asphalt parking lot, just over 27,000 gallons of water would run off.

The Heal the Planet Farm is 320 acres. So if we had a two-inch rain, and the landscape absorbed one inch of rain but the other inch ran off, we calculate that 9 million gallons of water would run off your property.

In your part of Southern Missouri, you have about 40 inches of rain per year. Every time there's a big heavy rain, I'd bet that half of it soaks into the land. The other half runs off.

We want to retain that rainwater, so the first thing we want to do is design a system to do just that.

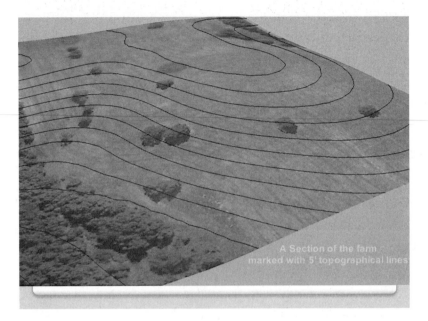

A Section of the farm marked with 5' topographical lines

In this view, the black lines represent a contour line. A contour line marks a specific elevation that is level across the landscape. Each one of these is 10 feet in elevation.

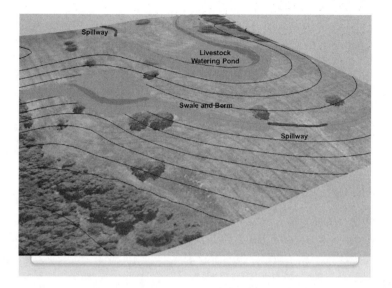

To help the plants get established, we put in a series of swales or ditches that follow the contours and fill up with water after a good rain allowing this captured water to slowly soak into the soil. We'll have a whole series of ponds as well that are filled by the swales too so that your cattle will always have plenty of water to drink.

If we get too much water, we must decide where we want the excess water to go. Once the pond is full of water, it spills out onto a ridge. You see that water is out in the open, rather than in the valley where it normally would go. When you have an excess of water going to a valley, you end up with a lot of erosion.

With this swale system, we have a lot of control over *where* we hold water, *how* we hold it, and *when we decide* to let it escape the system.

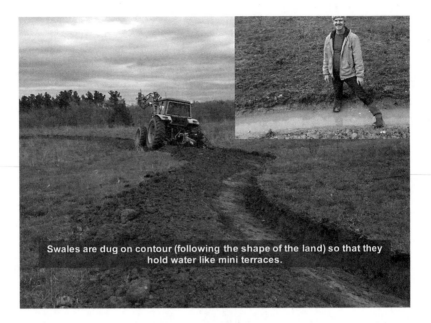

Swales are dug on contour (following the shape of the land) so that they hold water like mini terraces.

This is what we started doing on Heal the Planet Farm. Kevin is on the tractor, and the inset photo is of Adam standing in the water. He and I marked all the contours, and Kevin came in with a tractor and cut the swales in the land. A few days later, it rained hard. That's all water that would have been off the property if we had not cut those swales in.

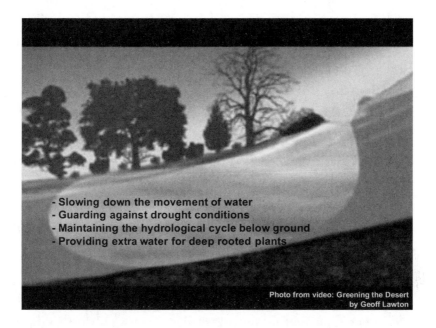

- Slowing down the movement of water
- Guarding against drought conditions
- Maintaining the hydrological cycle below ground
- Providing extra water for deep rooted plants

Photo from video: Greening the Desert
by Geoff Lawton

Here's what happens when we hold water on the landscape. Water gets a chance to rest, sit still, and slowly soak into the ground. The idea behind this design is to hold water—and thus fertility—high in the landscape for as long as possible. The water slowly soaks into the ground instead of running off the property.

Anything we plant downhill from the swale—any kind of a plant with a deep root system—can access this water once that system is charged. Typically, it takes four to six years to fully charge the subsoils of a poorly managed farm.

Once the land is rehydrated, there's so much water in the soils that you can grow for generations and never worry about drought. The permaculture concept here is to slow, spread and soak water into the ground.

Jordan: That's keeping it simple—slow, spread, and sink. Prior to embarking on our project together, we were losing quite a bit of water due to compacted soil and a lack of organic matter in the topsoil.

This is a fairly obvious observation, but water will always find the lowest point, and certainly on the 320 hilly acres of the Heal the Planet Farm, whenever there's a big rain, the outflow is absolutely huge.

I've heard it said that water is the Earth's most important resource, and the only capital that we should be thinking about for our future is biological capital. That biological capital is really soil organic matter—topsoil—and it could be the greatest inheritance we pass on to future generations because as important as water is, water does no good unless there is soil organic matter to hold it.

Bill: I wholeheartedly agree. What we're talking about here are four major elements that we find on this planet—water, air, sun, and earth. All four are essential and so important. But the plants are the great alchemists. They take these four basic elements and turn them into life. It's really the plants and trees that create security and abundance on this planet.

Let's say you have all the money in the world and can go to the moon. But what do you have? No air, no plants. It's really the plants that make it possible for the animal kingdom to survive and experience a sense of security and abundance, and healthy soil creates the plants. It all starts with the soil.

Now plants can grow, and once you've got a secure plant system, humans can sustainably harvest from that system. We can develop systems that are much more productive than nature would normally provide because we're designing them for us as humans, whereas nature might design it more for wildlife, for every insect, for every rodent, and for every bug. We're designing systems that still take care of all of that, but we can actually do better than nature does and create more abundance for wildlife and for ourselves.

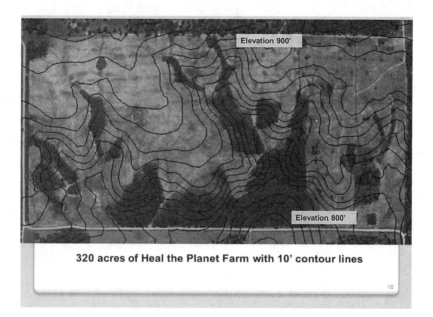

320 acres of Heal the Planet Farm with 10' contour lines

Jordan: Here we see the entire Heal the Planet Farm with contour lines for every ten-foot change in elevation.

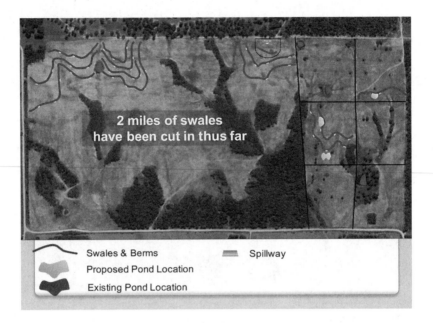

And here's where we are today with two miles of swales. We've also followed another recommendation of yours, Bill, and that is to "keyline" the property where we can. We know that plowing or the traditional tilling of the soil breaks up and can destroy microorganisms or underground ecology, and that's not something we want to do.

But "keylining" the soil with a Yeomans plow, invented by P.A. Yeomans of Australia, has done wonders for our land. We've found that the Yeomans plow has been one of the most valuable tools in permaculture.

Bill: In the 1950s, P.A. Yeomans, a mining engineer, gained custody of a 400 acre farm in Australia. He could see that his land was parched and losing water. As a mining hydrologist he knew there had to be *a way to hold water on the landscape.*

He came up with this idea of producing a version of subsoil plow that creates a thin cut and a below-the-ground furrow. He would then run this keyline plow on contour so that when rainwater fell, the excess would fill up the furrows thus holding thousands of extra gallons on the landscape, hydrating the soil.

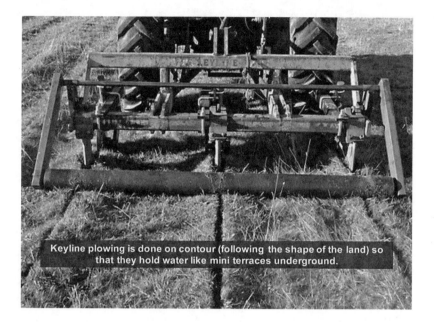

Keyline plowing is done on contour (following the shape of the land) so that they hold water like mini terraces underground.

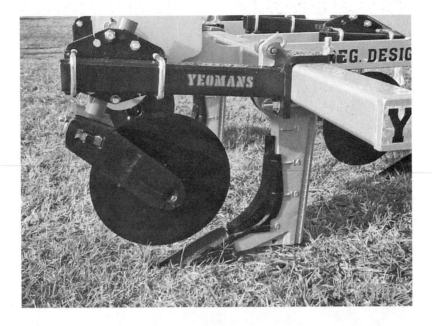

Over a period of five to ten years, P.A. Yeomans worked his entire farm using this keyline plow method. The neighbors laughed at him wondering what this city boy was trying to do.

The story goes that several years later, there was a three-year drought. Everything was brown everywhere except for one spot on the landscape, P.A. Yeoman's farm.

And all of a sudden, people got interested.

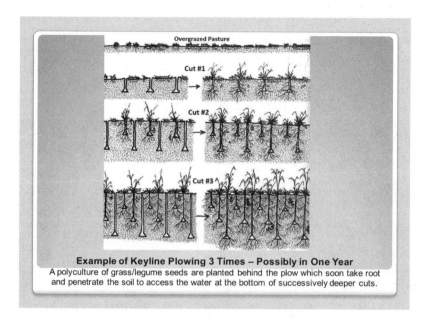

Example of Keyline Plowing 3 Times – Possibly in One Year
A polyculture of grass/legume seeds are planted behind the plow which soon take root and penetrate the soil to access the water at the bottom of successively deeper cuts.

The top of this image shows what a dormant, overgrazed pasture might look like after livestock have nibbled on the forage for some time. At your farm, Jordan, we're going down five or six inches with the keyline plow. Then right behind the plow we're sprinkling seeds that have a deep root system. Then 4-6 months later we'll come in again, offset the plow from the first cuts and go a bit deeper with the second pass. When the soil is broken up but not turned, the roots have a place to go, and the plants grow to be more lush.

Another tool we utilize at the Heal the Planet Farm is changing from set grazing—which means that livestock walk around and nibble wherever they want in a large fenced in area—to a holistic grazing system also called "ultra-high density intensive grazing," which means we limit the area the livestock can graze in to a short period of time and have them come back to the same spot no more than once every three to six months.

When the livestock return, the pasture is two or three feet high instead of the normal four or five inches high. They eat the grasses, legumes, herbs, and forbs, leave their fertilizer behind, and the next time it rains, the pasture becomes even more productive.

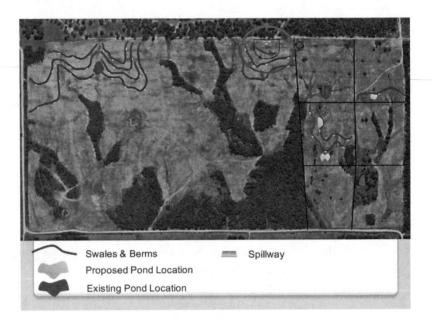

Swales & Berms	Spillway
Proposed Pond Location	
Existing Pond Location	

Jordan: One thing I wanted at the Heal the Planet Farm was a place where anyone can come and see what we're doing and seeking to accomplish in a "heal the planet" type of way.

The area circled in white is a "demonstration area" that we have set aside to highlight the permaculture principles in practice at the Heal the Planet Farm.

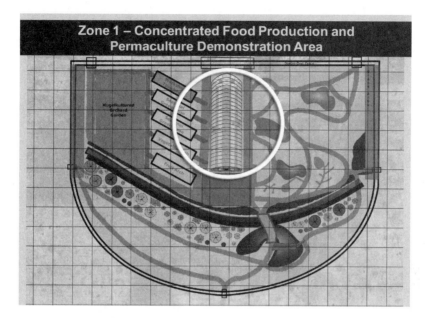

Zone 1 – Concentrated Food Production and Permaculture Demonstration Area

You can see that we will have a greenhouse as well as a path system so that people can walk around and see how plants can work together to become more productive.

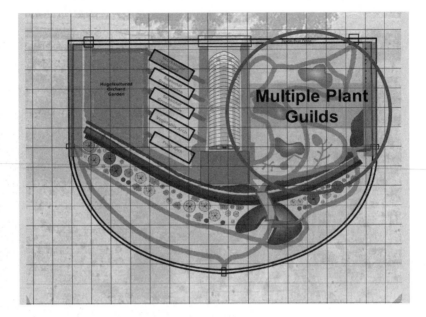

Bill: For instance, if we put three different kinds of plants in three different rows, they'd all do okay, but if we put them together in a precise way, all three of them could actually do better than if they were planted apart.

This is what is known as companion planting. You want to have plants that bring up nutrients; plants that fix nitrogen; plants with deep root systems that bring up moisture and share it; and plants that shade or nurse other plants. Plants working together.

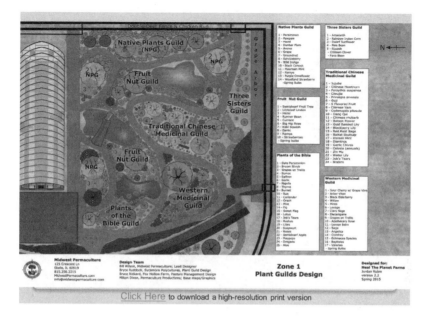

Click Here to download a high-resolution print version

To demonstrate this we've designed an area with various kind of plant communities or plant guilds. We'll have several areas that will focus on vegetables, herbs, and spices as well as guilds for fruits and nuts.

And Jordan, because of the work you do with nutritionally intense foods, we came up with a couple of medicinal guilds—the Chinese medicinal guild and a standard Western medicinal guild. We also designed a guild containing many plants that are mentioned in the Bible that have many health and healing properties. The Three Sisters' guild is a fun guild—corn, squash, and beans, and I know how passionate you are about high-antioxidant corn and various legumes with medicinal properties.

When our guild system is done, people can walk around and be quite inspired. This will be a highly functional landscape that is designed to support all kinds of plants. There will be annual plants mixed in with perennial plants. Everything will be quite beautiful.

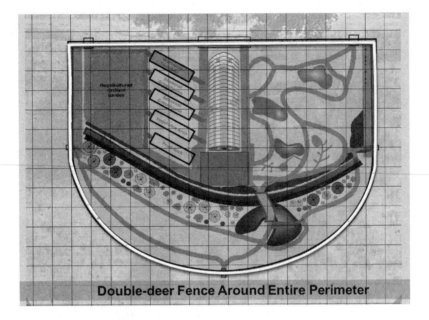

Double-deer Fence Around Entire Perimeter

Jordan: I know as soon as we started talking about this demonstration area that we had to discuss what to do about the deer. We have more deer on our property than we have livestock, as our acreage is home to thousands of whitetail. People all around Missouri call this part of the state a "whitetail haven." But we want to keep the deer from consuming our small plants. Sometimes they're real pests.

Bill: Deer are a problem in a lot of places, so we've designed in a "double deer fence." You can see on the slide that the line in white is where we need some sort of fencing to keep deer out.

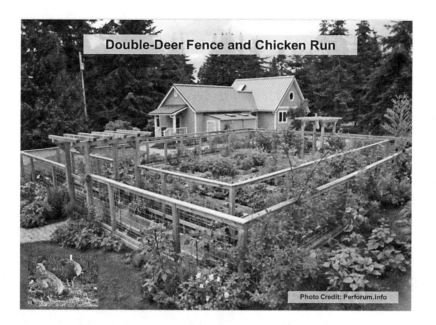

Double-Deer Fence and Chicken Run

Photo Credit: Perforum.info

Bill: We know that deer can hop a seven-foot fence rather easily. So instead of erecting a really tall fence around the entire property, which would give the demonstration area the feel of a state penitentiary, we will build a double deer fence where both fences are only four or five feet high but they're separated by a four-to-five foot space. We've learned that when deer come up to the edge of a double fence and can't see where to land clearly—their depth perception apparently is not all that acute—they won't try to jump it.

Another key concept in permaculture design is the idea of stacking functions. In other words, you ask yourself, "How many benefits can I get by adding this one feature?"

We see multiple functions for this fenced-in area, the first using this space between the fencing as a chicken run. That's one benefit, but guess what? Any insects, bugs, or rodents that want to come in and eat plants inside the garden have to get through that fence. When they try, the chickens will be there to gobble them up. Anything that creeps or crawls will get picked up by the chickens. They'll even jump and harvest bugs right out of the air.

We've learned from others who have a double deer fence with chickens in the corridor, and they had a 60 percent drop in insect pressure. So by putting in the double deer fence, we keep the deer out, keep chickens in, and keep the insect pressure down. The corridor fencing also protects chickens from predators such as hawks.

Notice the arch in this slide. On that arch, we can grow grapes. The grapes grow, and any excess grapes that drop on the ground become chicken feed. The arch also makes it difficult for hawks to swoop in and kill the chickens.

So with one simple structure—a double fence—we're getting quite a few different yields from it. We're trying to incorporate that kind of thinking throughout the Heal the Planet Farm.

Jordan: Adding chickens is a brilliant touch. Fowl are adept at eating ticks and flies. But chickens eat a lot more than bugs. When we moved two of our chicken houses, two field mice jumped out, and the chickens ran, caught, and ate them!

When chickens consume insects, those insects provide a superior source of calcium in their exoskeletons, as well as amazing sources of fat and phospholipids.

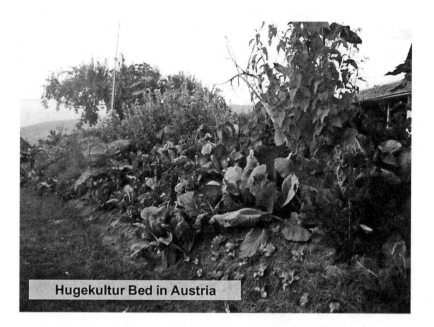

Hugekultur Bed in Austria

Probably my favorite word in permaculture is of European descent, and it's *hugelkultur*. I love unique and sophisticated terms that hardly anyone knows the meaning of. Makes me feel like an insider.

Bill: Hugelkultur is a German word for *mound culture.* In the Alpine regions of Germany and Austria, as you move up in elevation in the mountains to where the forest is dense, the soil is sparse—with rock underneath! And so you can't put in a traditional deep-bed garden of any kind.

People who lived in those areas hundreds of years ago realized that if they found a sunny opening in the forest, moved a few fallen logs into the space, and covered them with as much soil as they could find, they could create a raised planting bed or mound.

The trillions of beneficial microbes in the soil love it because they need food and shelter, and the log becomes that for them. As the bacteria count explodes inside the hugelkultur beds, there's more nutrition for plants.

The Heal the Planet Farm demonstration area will include hugelkultur beds, and they're perfect for soil that's been depleted. Once the hugelkultur is in, we'll plant annual crops or herbs on the berm. Next to the berm will be a variety of trees.

Hugelkultur does break down over time. After fifteen or twenty years, the wood eventually deteriorates to the point where the pile becomes insignificant. My wife took this picture when we were in Austria.

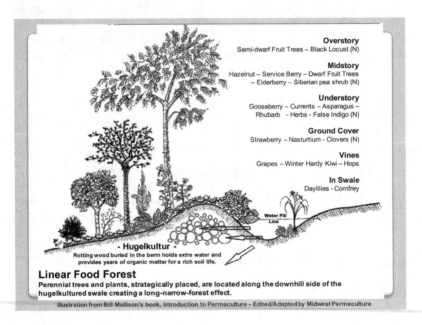

Overstory
Semi-dwarf Fruit Trees – Black Locust (N)

Midstory
Hazelnut – Service Berry – Dwarf Fruit Trees – Elderberry – Siberian pea shrub (N)

Understory
Gooseberry – Currents – Asparagus – Rhubarb - Herbs - False Indigo (N)

Ground Cover
Strawberry – Nasturtium - Clovers (N)

Vines
Grapes – Winter Hardy Kiwi – Hops

In Swale
Daylilies - Comfrey

Water Fill Line

- Hugelkultur -
Rotting wood buried in the berm holds extra water and provides years of organic matter for a rich soil life.

Linear Food Forest
Perennial trees and plants, strategically placed, are located along the downhill side of the hugelkultured swale creating a long-narrow-forest effect.

Illustration from Bill Mollison's book, Introduction to Permaculture – Edited/Adapted by Midwest Permaculture

This slide shows a cross section of the swale, the hugelkultur, and then short-rooted plants on top of the hugelkultur. Notice the trees are planted next to the hugelkultur, not on it. Some the roots from any trees will make their way to the hugelkultur to access the nutrients but we don't want the tree hanging in mid-air when the pile breaks down to almost nothing over the years.

You can see that by digging a swale, we can use that dirt to cover the rotting logs. It all works together.

Jordan: This is truly amazing. If you look at our current land, not just the 320 acres but also our nearly 4,000 contiguous acres, we have loads of trees. When a tree has fallen, it begins to form its own hugelkultur mound over time. It's like someone's trash can truly become someone else's treasure. And I'll add this too, in a German way: what would be really cool is to take a hugelkultur mound, plant cabbage on top, and then make sauerkraut. So then we can have a double-cultured sauerkraut thing going.

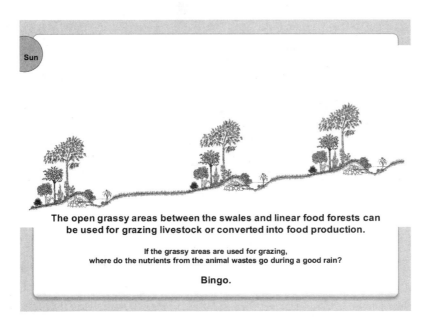

The open grassy areas between the swales and linear food forests can be used for grazing livestock or converted into food production.

If the grassy areas are used for grazing, where do the nutrients from the animal wastes go during a good rain?

Bingo.

Bill: Notice the series of hugelkultur swales using the contour of the land. We can plant right next to the swale and have cattle grazing on the grassland in between the trees. When the cows leave, they leave all their fertility behind, and the next time it rains, where does all that fertility wash to? It washes right down to the next swale, where the nutrients lock in for the plants as quickly as they can absorb them.

We're doing several things here: we're slowing water down, we're holding water, we're feeding cattle, and we're letting plants use their waste to generate material for the entire landscape, and we're feeding wildlife, livestock and ourselves.

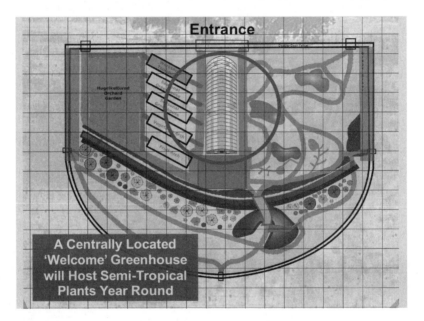

Jordan: You can see the area on the left where we're going to have a hugelkultur garden and orchard. I'm just as excited about our greenhouse, which is loosely inspired by my favorite ride at the Epcot theme park at Disney World—the "Living with the Land" ride, which is a slow-moving boat cruise through multimedia agricultural displays and four working greenhouses.

Our greenhouse won't be as elaborate, of course, but visitors will have a great experience and see how we're heating and cooling the greenhouse through several "regenerative" practices.

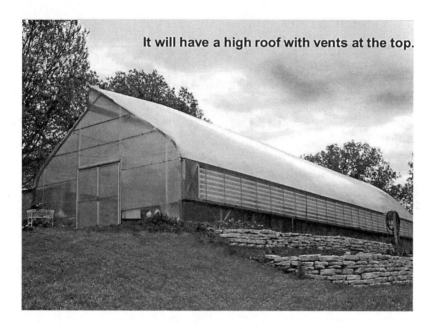

It will have a high roof with vents at the top.

Bill: Our challenge in designing a greenhouse for Missouri is not how to keep it warm in the winter but how to keep from burning up in the middle of the blazing hot summers.

We know the earth beneath our feet is temperate year round—around 55 degrees. What if we were able to pull that 55 degree air into the greenhouse?

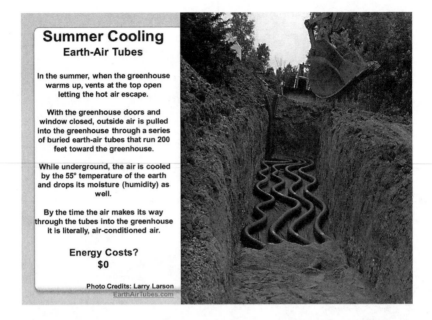

Here's a system of "earth air tubes" that takes air from the ground and cools the greenhouse. This image shows how the tubes are placed in a trench, and the air entering the greenhouse basically becomes air-conditioned or air-cooled. We'll have cool 55 degree air coming into a greenhouse that could reach temperatures on a hot sunny day of 140 degrees if we kept it closed up.

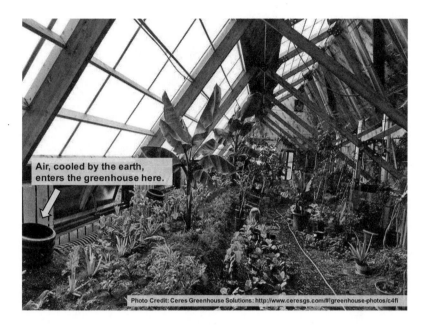

You can see how the cooler air will come into the greenhouse through the larger pipe to the left. The Phipps Conservatory in Pittsburgh, Pennsylvania uses this exact type of system.

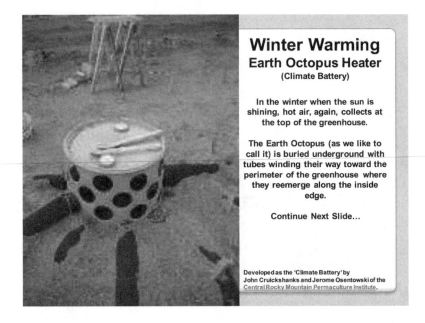

Winter Warming
Earth Octopus Heater
(Climate Battery)

In the winter when the sun is shining, hot air, again, collects at the top of the greenhouse.

The Earth Octopus (as we like to call it) is buried underground with tubes winding their way toward the perimeter of the greenhouse where they reemerge along the inside edge.

Continue Next Slide...

Developed as the 'Climate Battery' by John Cruickshanks and Jerome Osentowski of the Central Rocky Mountain Permaculture Institute.

But what do we do in the wintertime? This Earth Octopus, which was developed by Jerome Osentowski at the Central Rocky Mountain Permaculture Institute, connects to a pipe that runs up to the top of the greenhouse, where the warm air always rises to. That warm air is then sucked down into the drum and pushed under the greenhouse through the earth where the heat is absorbed by the soil. It's ingenious, really.

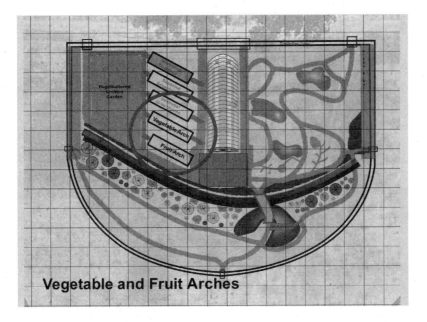

Vegetable and Fruit Arches

On the other side of the greenhouse, we'll put in two structures to demonstrate how beautiful the growing of fruits and vegetables can be.

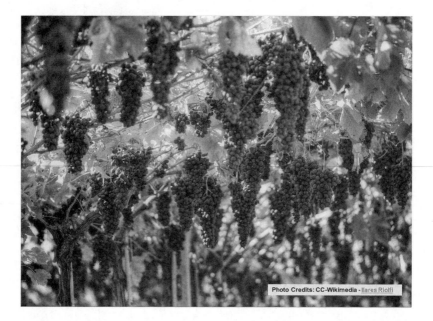

Photo Credits: CC-Wikimedia - Ilares Riolfi

This is a grape arbor attached to a beautiful arch that provides wonderful shade during the summer time protecting fruit and people from the sun and wind. In the wintertime, all the leaves fall off, which gives you bends of sunlight.

This is another example of permaculture design, but the big picture is that we want to repair soils and our ecosystem. We've done a lot of damage to this planet, but permaculture is a way to provide for ourselves and take care of the planet. We also want to assure abundance for future generations.

The good news is that nature will work with us. Nature wants us to win. All we have to do is put these systems into place, and nature takes over.

Jordan: With permaculture, we can reverse the curse of degeneration. Bill, I'm a huge fan of the work you and Midwest Permaculture are doing. My hope is that by giving you a blank canvas at the Heal the Planet Farm, you can paint the greatest permaculture picture that exists today. Even if our 320 acres within 4,000 acres is a drop in the bucket in terms of what needs to be done, the good news is we're starting with a place that has a unique climate with extreme highs and extreme lows and little fertility in the soil. We feel like we're the New York, New York of agriculture: if we can make it there, we'll make it anywhere. We're thrilled to be partnering with you on the Heal the Planet Farm project.

Our first permaculture design course took place in October 2015, and was such a great success. Looking ahead, our goal is to invite people from all over the world to come and learn about how they can bring the art and the science of permaculture to their own backyard or farm. For more information on our Permaculture Design Courses, visit www .GetRealNutrition/PermacultureDesign.

If you ever attend a permaculture course at the Heal the Planet Farm, conducted by Midwest Permaculture, you will play a role in the development of the Heal the Planet Farm. Our goal is to increase the fertility of our soil five to tenfold in the next five years.

Let me close by sharing my vision for the Heal the Planet Farm:

1. We want to sustainably feed those who are part of the mission.

We have a team responsible for caring for the land, the animals, and the plants. Our goal for our employees and interns is to allow them to reap the fruits of their labor so they can consume the foods that they have a part in growing—and live in a sustainable way.

For those who live and work on the Heal the Planet Farm, wanting to consume fresh food is part of their passion. Obviously, we can't grow year-round outdoors in Missouri, but we will have constant indoor growing. There are also ways to preserve the foods with canning, drying, and of course fermentation—all the methods our ancestors used. We also want to feed those who come to the Heal the Planet Farm for the permaculture design courses that will train the next generation of organic farmers, which we'll have four to six times a year.

2. We want to grow ingredients that comprise our consumer products.

For example, there are certain crops we are growing right now called velvet bean (*mucuna pruriens*) that have very powerful nutritional compounds to be used in future product formulations. They are very hard to find domestically and almost impossible to find organic. So we're growing them plus a novel strain of high-antioxidant purple corn. We also have multiple herbs and spices that we're growing. We will use ingredients grown on the Heal the Planet Farm in our Get Real Nutrition formulations.

3. We want the nutrients we create on the Heal the Planet Farm to help feed the local community.

This is where the Heal the Planet Foundation comes in. Our goal is to take the foods that we produce—animal and plant foods—and feed the local communities, partnering with various local nonprofit organizations.

We're located in Koshkonong, Missouri, a sparsely populated community of just over two hundred persons. The average income is $16,000 per family, significantly lower than the national average of $50,052.

While people in the Ozarks may not appreciate all the foods that we're growing, we're going to help families consume some of the world's healthiest foods coming from the Heal the Planet Farm, which we feel will accomplish the goals set forth in this book. That's really what the

Heal the Planet Foundation is about—healing the planet's skin (soil) and its residents (people).

Perhaps you want to get involved with us. You can come to one of our permaculture design certificate (PDC) courses, which last only eight to ten days thanks to the pre-training materials we also provide all students. The internationally recognized PDC Course is an amazing opportunity to learn how to practice the principles of permaculture and healing the planet, whether you have a small backyard or a large farm. We want to do our part to train the next generation of eco-regenerative, beyond-organic farmers.

You can even become an intern. We'll be inviting some of the top permaculture design students to stay and assist us at Heal the Planet Farm. And then some of our interns will go to other farms, or perhaps start their own farms, or maybe they'll travel around the world teaching these principles. And some will stay and become employees at the Heal the Planet Farm.

You can support the Heal the Planet Foundation, where we are not only testing these principles in action on our 320 acres, but we are helping educate other organizations to do the same thing.

Remember, live in such a way that you leave the planet in better condition than you found it, and the planet and its people will heal itself.

Source Material

INTRODUCTION: THE REVOLUTION OF REGENERATION

"We're losing more and more of it every day," said David Montgomery…from Tom Paulson, "The Lowdown on Dirt: It's Disappearing," *Seattle Post-Intelligencer*, January 21, 2008, http://www.seattlepi.com/national/article/The-lowdown-on-topsoil-It-s-disappearing-1262214.php.

"Take cancer for starters…" from "Lifetime Risk of Developing or Dying from Cancer," American Cancer Society, October 1, 2014, http://www.cancer.org/cancer/cancerbasics/lifetime-probability-of-developing-or-dying-from-cancer.

1: THE CIRCLE OF LIFE: REAL NUTRIENTS FROM REAL FOODS CREATE REAL HEALTH

"According to the Gallup Gardening Survey…" from Kathy LaLiberte, "Fertilizer Basics," Gardeners Supply, accessed July 26, 2015, http://www.gardeners.com/how-to/fertilizer-basics/5161.html.

"Compared to the old stone methods…" from "What's Wrong with Modern Wheat?" Grainstorm, accessed July 26, 2015, http://www.grainstorm.com/pages/rant.

"No one was asking that question because the American Medical Association's
Council of Foods and Nutrition and the Council on Pharmacy and
Chemistry issued a statement in 1938…" from "Celebrating 70 Years of
Enrichment," Northeast Foods, accessed July 26, 2015, http://nefoods
.com/pdf/70-Years-of-Enrichment.pdf.

2: SPROUTING TO LIFE

"In the late 1990s, research teams at Johns Hopkins…" from Natalie Angier,
"Researchers Find a Concentrated Anticancer Substance in Broccoli
Sprouts," *The New York Times*, September 15, 1997, http://www.nytimes
.com/1997/09/16/us/researchers-find-a-concentrated-anticancer-substance
-in-broccoli-sprouts.html.

"And then in 2014, Johns Hopkins announced that results…" from "Chemical
Derived from Broccoli Sprouts Shows Promise in Treating Autism,"
Johns Hopkins Medicine, October 13, 2014, http://www
.hopkinsmedicine.org/news/media/releases/chemical_derived_from
_broccoli_sprouts_shows_promise_in_treating_autism.

3: FANTASTIC FERMENTATION

"That's a good thing because food scraps make up 20 percent to 30
percent…" from Kaye Spector, "How to Compost in Your Apartment,"
EcoWatch, December 16, 2013, http://ecowatch.com/2013/12/16/
how-to-compost-apartment/.

"In 2012, the most recent year for which estimates are available, American
tossed more than 35 millions tons of food…." from Roberto A.
Ferdman, "Americans Throw out More Food than Plastic, Paper,
Metal, and Glass," *Washington Post*, September 23, 2014, http://www
.washingtonpost.com/blogs/wonkblog/wp/2014/09/23/americans-throw
-out-more-food-than-plastic-paper-metal-or-glass/.

"In 2014, thirty-nine of California's fifty-eight counties shipped more than 5
percent of their trash and recycling materials…" from Jessica Garrison,
"Central Valley Residents Tire of Receiving L.A.'s Urban Waste," *Los
Angeles Times*, November 25, 2012, http://articles.latimes.com/2012
/nov/25/local/la -me-central-valley-20121126.

"The Greek philosopher Aristotle praised…." from Dana Terebelski and Nancy Ralph, "Pickle History Timeline," NY Food Museum, accessed July 30, 2015, http://www.nyfoodmuseum.org/_ptime.htm.

"Lactic acid is a natural preservative that inhibits putrefying bacteria…" from Sally Fallon et al., *Nourishing Traditions: The Cookbook That Challenges Politically Correct Nutrition and the Diet Dictocrats* (Brandywine, MD: NewTrends Pub., 2001), 89.

"Ophiocordyceps sinensis became famous in the U.S. based on its use by the Chinese women athletes…" from D.C. Steinkraus and J.B. Whitfield, "Chinese Caterpillar Fungus and World Record Runners," *American Entomologist* 40, no. 4 (1994): 235-239, doi:10.1093/ae/40.4.235.

"What's not up for debate is how Ophiocordyceps sinensis has been described as a medicine in Chinese and Tibetan traditional health volumes…" from Ashokkumar Panda and Kailashchandra Swain, "Traditional Uses and Medicinal Potential of Cordyceps Sinensis of Sikkim," *Journal of Ayurveda and Integrative Medicine J Ayurveda Integr Med* 2, no. 1 (2011): 9-13, doi:10.4103/0975-9476.78183.

"Trametes Versicolor is the botanical name for the turkey tail mushroom…" from Paul Stamets, "Turkey Tail Mushrooms Help Immune System Fight Cancer," The Huffington Post, October 26, 2012, http://www.huffingtonpost.com/paul-stamets/mushrooms-cancer_b_1560691.html.

"But the latest research made headlines in 2015: scientists at the Chang Gung University in Taiwan…" from Lizzie Parry, "Could Mushrooms Be the Key to Losing Weight?" Daily Mail Online, June 24, 2015, http://www.dailymail.co.uk/health/article-3137253/Could-MUSHROOMS-key-losing-weight-Fungi-used-Chinese-medicine-alters-gut-bacteria-used-treat-obesity.html.

"Lion's mane mushrooms are increasingly studied…" from Paul Stamets, "Lion's Mane: A Mushroom That Improves Your Memory and Mood?" *The Huffington Post*, October 8, 2012, http://www.huffingtonpost.com/paul-stamets/mushroom-memory_b_1725583.html.

4: EAT ORGANIC

"For shoppers, a green-and-white USDA Organic seal on single-ingredient foods like meat, eggs, and cheese…" from Peter Laufer, "Five Myths about Organic Food," *Washington Post,* June 20, 2014, http://www.washingtonpost.com/opinions/five-myths-about-organic-food/2014/06/20/43d23f14-f566-11e3-a3a5-42be35962a52_story.html.

"In India in 1945, at war's end, malaria infected an estimated 75 million…" from Vincent Landon, "DDT: From Miracle Chemical to Banned Pollutant," Swiss Info Magazine, May 3, 2003, http://www.swissinfo.ch/eng/ddt--from-miracle-chemical-to-banned-pollutant/3253684.

"A full-page advertisement in Time magazine in 1947…" from Joe Debrow, "When Did We Start Using So Many Pesticides? The Important Backstory…," Rodale's Organic Life, accessed July 31, 2015, http://www.rodalenews.com/when-did-we-start-using-pesticides.

"The U.S. Environmental Protection Agency (EPA) had this to say…" from "Human Health Issues," EPA, October 17, 2014, http://www.epa.gov/pesticides/health/human.htm.

"The majority of soybean, corn, canola, and sunflower seeds planted in the U.S. are sprayed with neonicotinoid pesticides…" from Dr. Joseph Mercola, "US Honeybee Losses Soar Over Last Year," Mercola.com, May 26, 2015, http://articles.mercola.com/sites/articles/archive/2015/05/26/honeybee-losses.aspx?e_cid=20150526Z1_DNL_art_2&utm_source=dnl&utm_medium=email&utm_content=art2&utm_campaign=20150526Z1&et_cid=DM75683&et_rid=967090335.

"A Harvard study released in 2014 reported that there…" from Mark J. Miller, "U.S. Honeybee Losses Not as Severe This Year," National Geographic, May 15, 2014, accessed July 31, 2015, http://news.nationalgeographic.com/news/2014/05/140515-honeybees-pesticides-usda-pollinators-food.

"The difference between organic and conventional produce was so striking…" from David Gutierrez, "Huge New Study Proves Organic Foods Are Healthier and More Nutritious," NaturalNews, July 16, 2014, http://www.naturalnews.com/046024_organic_food_nutritional_content_pesticide_residue.html.

"Jared Stone, author of Year of the Cow..." from Jared Stone, "Why Grass-Fed Cattle Are Better," Los Angeles Times, May 20, 2015, http://www.latimes.com/opinion/op-ed/la-oe-stone-drought-grass-fed-beef-20150520-story.html.

"Alan Savory, a biologist and former member of the Rhodesian Parliament..." from Allan Savory, "How to Fight Desertification and Reverse Climate Change," TED, March 2013, http://www.ted.com/talks/allan_savory_how_to_green_the_world_s_deserts_and_reverse_climate_change/transcript?language=en.

"A thirty-year study by the Rodale Institute..." from Max Follmer, "30-Year Study Proves It: Organic Farming Is Best," TakePart, October 5, 2011, http://www.takepart.com/article/2011/10/05/30-year-study-proves-it-organic-farming-best.

"In another study published in The Journal of Applied Nutrition..." from "Organic Food Is More Nutritious Than Conventional Food," *Journal of Applied Nutrition*, 1993, accessed July 31, 2015, http://www.organicconsumers.org/Organic/organicstudy.cfm.

5: SAY NO TO GMO

"A nationwide survey released by researchers at Rutgers University found..." from "Most Americans Pay Little Attention to Genetically Modified Foods, Survey Says," Rutgers Today, November 1, 2013, http://news.rutgers.edu/research-news/most-americans-pay-little-attention-genetically-modified-foods-survey -says/20131101.

"You just can't get an elephant to mate with a corn plant..." from Sasha Nemecek, "Does the World Needs Gm Foods?" *Scientific American* 284, no. 4 (2001): 39, doi:10.1038/scientificamerican0401-62.

"A meta-analysis, which reviewed 147 other studies..." from "Why Some Farmers Choose to Grow GMO Crops," Capital Press, January 29, 2015, http://www.capitalpress.com/Opinion/Editorials/20150129/why-some-farmers-choose-to-grow-gmo-crops.

"We all know stories of tobacco, asbestos, and DDT…" from Jeffrey Smith, "State of the Science on the Health Risks of GM Foods," Centers for Responsible Technology, accessed July 31, 2015, http://www .responsibletechnology.org/docs/145.pdf.

"Today the vast majority of foods in supermarkets contain genetically modified substances…" from "Should We Grow GM Crops?" PBS, accessed July 31, 2015, http://www.pbs.org/wgbh/harvest/exist/arguments.html.

"The Non-GMO Project, an independent organization, has stepped…" from "GMO Facts," The NonGMO Project, accessed July 31, 2015, http:// www.nongmoproject.org/learn-more/.

"Corn is what feeds the steer that becomes your steak…" from Michael Pollan, qtd. in "Why Is Corn in Everything?" This Conscious Life, June 21, 2011, http://thisconsciouslife.com/2011/06/21/why -is-corn-in-everything/.

"The FDA concluded that 'these foods are safe and nutritious as their conventional counterparts…'" from Elizabeth Whitman, "GMO Apples and Potatoes Approved by FDA; Labeling Not Required," International Business Times, March 20, 2015, http://www.ibtimes.com/ gmo-apples-potatoes-approved-fda-labeling-not-required-1854280.

"Scientists at the University of Maryland and the U.S. Department of Agriculture believe…" from Todd Woody, "Scientists Discover What's Killing the Bees and It's Worse than You Thought," Quartz, July 25, 2013, http://qz.com/107970/scientists-discover -whats-killing-the-bees-and-its-worse-than-you-thought/.

6: GO GLUTEN-FREE

"I had started to feel really lethargic…" from Drew Brees, "Drew Brees on Living Without Dairy," Whole Foods, October 20, 2013, http://www .wholefoodsmarket.com/blog/drew-brees-living-without-dairy.

"Unless the cyclists love what they're eating…" from Alastair Bland, "The Epic 2,200-Mile Tour De France Is Also a Test of Epic Eating," NPR, July 23, 2014, http://www.npr.org/blogs/thesalt/2014/07/23/334423902/ the-epic-2-200-mile-tour-de-france-is-also-a-test-of-epic-eating.

"Dr. Cetojevic had a feeling he knew what was ailing his fellow Serb…" from Paul Newman, "Revealed: The Diet That Saved Novak Djokovic," The Independent, August 19, 2013, accessed July 31, 2015, http://www.independent.co.uk/sport/tennis/revealed-the-diet-that-saved-novak-djokovic-8775333.html.

"Nutritionally speaking, gluten is useless…" from Anna Medaris Miller, "Many Athletes Tout the Gluten-free Way. What's the Science behind the Claim?" Washington Post, October 14, 2013, http://www.washingtonpost.com/national/health-science/many-athletes-tout-the-gluten-free-way-whats-the-science-behind-the-claim/2013/10/14/cc0b601c-d42f-11e2-b05f-3ea3f0e7bb5a_story.html.

7: THE POWER OF PLANTS

"A University of Illinois at Urbana-Champaign study on the effects of blueberries on prostate cancer…" from Amy Boulanger, "Health Benefits of Blueberries: 5 Reasons to Eat More Blueberries," Medical Daily, June 12, 2013, http://www.medicaldaily.com/health-benefits-blueberries-5-reasons-eat-more-blueberries -246727.

"Apples contain flavonoids such as quercetin, which can assist alpha-amylase…" from "What's New and Beneficial about Apples," Whole Foods, accessed July 31, 2015, http://www.whfoods.com/genpage.php?tname=foodspice&dbid=15.

"In a health study of about 40,000 U.S. women, researchers analyzed their apple consumption…" from Karen Collins, "Apples Pack a Big Antioxidant Punch," NBC News, January 19, 2007, http://www.nbcnews.com/id/16678580/ns/health-diet_and_nutrition/.

"Hailed as a superfood and a rising superstar, kale has seen a 400 percent increase…" from "The Rise and Rise of Kale," Blue Apron Blog, November 19, 213, http://blog.blueapron.com/the-rise-and-rise-of-kale/.

"I was a freshman in high school when President G.W. Bush…" from Maureen Dowd, "I'm President, So No More Broccoli!" The New York Times, March 22, 1990, http://www.nytimes.com/1990/03/23/us/i-m-president-so-no-more-broccoli.html.

"Let me say this," the President responded…from David Jackson, "Obama: I Really Do Eat Broccoli," USA Today, August 07, 2013, http://www.usatoday.com/story/theoval/2013/08/07/obama-jay-leno-broccoli-michelle-obama/2627037/.

"Beets contain high amounts of boron…" from Kiley Dumas, "6 Health Benefits of Eating Beets," Good Food Life, May 20, 2012, http://www.fullcircle.com/goodfoodlife/2012/05/10/6-health-benefits-of-eating-beets/.

"According to the virtual World Carrot Museum, Greek physician Pedanius Dioscorides…" from "History of the Carrot Part III," World Carrot Museum, accessed July 31, 2015, http://www.carrotmuseum.co.uk/history2.html.

"Researchers at the U.S. Department of Agriculture found that study participants who consumed two carrots per day…" from "Carrot Sayings, Quotes, Fun Facts, and Trivia," Koffee Klatch Gals, October 14, 2014, http://koffeeklatchgals.hubpages.com/hub/Carrot-sayings-quotes-fun-facts-and-trivia.

"Researchers at William Patterson University in New Jersey…" from Lenny Bernstein, "Watercress Tops List of 'powerhouse Fruits and Vegetables.' Who Knew?" Washington Post, June 05, 2014, http://www.washingtonpost.com/news/to-your-health/wp/2014/06/05/finally-a-list-of-powerhouse-fruits-and-vegetables-ranked-by-how-much-nutrition-they-contain.

"A 2008 study in *Journal of the American Dietetic Association*…" from Amy Long Carrera, "Garbanzo Bean Health Benefits," Healthy Eating, accessed July 31, 2015, http://healthyeating.sfgate.com/garbanzo-bean-health-benefits-4264.html.

"Fifty different studies were released in 2012 and 2013…" from Case Adams, "Over 50 New Studies Prove Ashwagandha Can Treat a Myriad of Conditions," Heal Naturally, February 05, 2013, http://www.realnatural.org/over-fifty-recent-studies-prove-ashwagandhas-potential-for-treating-a-myriad-of-conditions/.

"A 2001 study published in the journal *Advances in Therapy* found that a garlic supplement can reduce the number of colds by 63 percent…" from Lizette Borreli, "7 Reasons You Should Eat More Garlic," Medical Daily, March 03, 2015, http://www.medicaldaily.com/garlic-good-you-7-surprising-benefits-garlic-optimal-health-324114.

"A 2005 study published in the Indian Journal of Physiology and Pharmacology…" Ibid.

8: AVOID EIGHT COMMON ALLERGENS

"Food allergies are certainly nothing to brush off…" from "About Food Allergies," from "About Food Allergies," Food Allergy Research & Education, accessed July 30, 2015, http://www.foodallergy.org/about -food-allergies.

"The smoke-and-mirrors approach is working…" from Janet Larsen and J. Matthew Roney, "Farmed Fish Production Overtakes Beef," EcoWatch, June 12, 2013, http://ecowatch.com/2013/06/12/ farmed-fish-production-overtakes-beef/.

"Soy is one of the more common food allergies…" from "Soy Allergy," Food Allergy Research & Education, accessed July 30, 2015, http://www .foodallergy.org/allergens/soy-allergy.

"So soy isn't really soy…" from Dr. Joseph Mercola, "Soy: This 'Beloved' Food Can Cause Allergic Reactions for Years—and Infertility for Generations!" Mercola.com, March 14, 2011, http://articles.mercola .com/sites/articles/archive/2011/03/14/is-the-hidden-soy-in-your-foods -contributing-to-illness.aspx.

9: BECOME AN ARTISANAL EATER

"The word *artisan* suggests that the product is less likely to be mass-produced…" from Bruce Horovitz, "Marketers Use Artisan Label to Evoke More Sales," *USA Today*, October 25, 2011, http:// usatoday30.usatoday.com/money/industries/food/story/2011-10-21/food -products-christened-artisan/50896420/1.

"The Hartman Group, a food and beverage consulting firm, says you should ask yourself three questions…" from Randy Bell, "Clearing up Confusion about Artisan Food," MSU Extension, May 30, 2013, http:// msue.anr.msu.edu/news/clear.

10: HEAL THE PLANET: LIVING THE ECO-REGENERATIVE LIFESTYLE

"The average American drinks 167 disposable water bottles each year…" from "Bottled Water Facts," Ban the Bottle, accessed July 30, 2015, http://www.banthebottle.net/bottled-water-facts/.

About Jordan Rubin

Jordan Rubin, one of America's most recognized and respected natural health experts, is founder and CEO of Get Real Nutrition.

Known as America's Biblical Health Coach, he is the *New York Times* best-selling author of *The Maker's Diet* and twenty-three additional health titles. An international motivational speaker and host of the weekly television show "Living Beyond Organic" that reaches over 30 million households worldwide, Jordan has lectured on natural health on five continents and forty-six states in the U.S.

Jordan founded Garden of Life, a leading whole-food nutritional supplement company, and Beyond Organic, a vertically integrated organic food and beverage company farming thousands of organic acres.

In 2015, Jordan started the Heal the Planet Farm, a regenerative permaculture retreat, and the Heal the Planet Foundation, a nonprofit effort to rebuild infertile soil and provide nutritious food for those in need.

Jordan's new company, Get Real Nutrition, was founded in 2015 to lead a revolution of regeneration in body, mind, and planet. He resides in Missouri, California, and Florida with his wife, Nicki, and their six children.

For more information on Get Real Nutrition,
please visit GetRealNutrition.com.

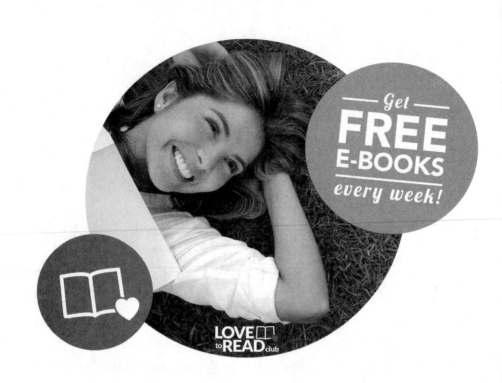